W.B. SAUNDERS COMPANY
A Division of Elsevier Inc.

1600 John F. Kennedy Boulevard • Suite 1800 • Philadelphia, Pennsylvania 19103-2899

http://www.vetexotic.theclinics.com

VETERINARY CLINICS OF NORTH AMERICA: EXOTIC ANIMAL PRACTICE Volume 13, Number 1
January 2010 ISSN 1094-9194, ISBN-13: 978-1-4377-1883-6

Editor: John Vassallo; j.vassallo@elsevier.com

Veterinary Clinics of North America: Exotic Animal Practice (ISSN 1094-9194) is published in January, May, and September by Elsevier, Inc., 360 Park Avenue South, New York, NY 10010-1710. Subscription prices are $198.00 per year for US individuals, $329.00 per year for US institutions, $103.00 per year for US students and residents, $234.00 per year for Canadian individuals, $388.00 per year for Canadian institutions, $264.00 per year for international individuals, $388.00 per year for international institutions and $132.00 per year for Canadian and foreign students/residents. To receive student/resident rate, orders must be accompanied by name of affiliated institution, date of term, and the *signature* of program/residency coordinator on institution letterhead. Orders will be billed at individual rate until proof of status is received. Foreign air speed delivery is included in all *Clinics* subscription prices. All prices are subject to change without notice. **POSTMASTER:** Send address changes to *Veterinary Clinics of North America: Exotic Animal Practice*, Elsevier Health Sciences Division, Subscription Customer Service, 3251 Riverport Lane, Maryland Heights, MO 63043. **Customer Service: Telephone: 1-800-654-2452** (U.S. and Canada); **1-314-447-8871** (outside U.S. and Canada). **Fax: 1-314-447-8029. E-mail: journalscustomerservice-usa@elsevier.com** (for print support); **journalsonlinesupport-usa@elsevier.com** (for online support).

Reprints. For copies of 100 or more of articles in this publication, please contact the Commercial Reprints Department, Elsevier Inc., 360 Park Avenue South, New York, New York 10010-1710. Tel.: (212)-633-3813; Fax: (212)-633-1935; E-mail: reprints@elsevier.com.

Veterinary Clinics of North America: Exotic Animal Practice is covered in *MEDLINE/PubMed (Index Medicus).*

Printed and bound by CPI Group (UK) Ltd, Croydon, CR0 4YY

Transferred to Digital Print 2011

Contributors

CONSULTING EDITOR

AGNES E. RUPLEY, DVM
Diplomate, American Board of Veterinary Practitioners—Avian Practice; and Director and
Chief Veterinarian, All Pets Medical and Laser Surgical Center, College Station, Texas

GUEST EDITORS

SHARMAN M. HOPPES, DVM
Diplomate, American Board of Veterinary Practitioners—Avian Practice; Clinical Associate
Professor, Zoological Medicine, Department of Veterinary Small Animal Clinical Sciences,
College of Veterinary Medicine and Biomedical Sciences, Texas A&M University,
College Station, Texas

PATRICIA GRAY, DVM, MS
Resident, Zoological Medicine/Schubot Exotic Bird Health Center, College of Veterinary
Medicine and Biomedical Sciences, Texas A&M University, College Station, Texas

AUTHORS

GERRY M. DORRESTEIN, DVM, PhD
Diplomate, Veterinary Pathology; Honorary Member European College of Avian Medicine
and Surgery, Diagnostic Pathology Laboratorium NOIVBD, Veldhoven, The Netherlands

VICKY L. HAINES, DVM
Diplomate, American College of Laboratory Animal Medicine; Associate Research
Scientist, Texas A&M Institute for Preclinical Studies; Adjunct Faculty Member,
Department of Veterinary Small Animal Clinical Sciences, College of Veterinary Medicine
and Biomedical Sciences, Texas A&M University, College Station, Texas

SHARMAN M. HOPPES, DVM
Diplomate, American Board of Veterinary Practitioners—Avian Practice; Clinical Associate
Professor, Zoological Medicine, Department of Veterinary Small Animal Clinical Sciences,
Texas A&M University, College of Veterinary Medicine and Biomedical Sciences,
College Station, Texas

JEFFREY R. JENKINS, DVM
Diplomate, American Board of Veterinary Practitioners—Avian Practice; Avian & Exotic
Animal Hospital Inc, San Diego, California

ANGELA M. LENNOX, DVM
Diplomate, American Board of Veterinary Practitioners—Avian Practice; Avian and Exotic
Animal Clinic, Indianapolis, Indiana

ANDREW M. LENTINI, PhD
Curatorial Keeper of Amphibians and Reptiles, Animal Health Centre, Toronto Zoo,
Scarborough, Ontario, Canada

conditions that arise with advancing age may involve various body systems including the musculoskeletal, cardiovascular, and others. Falconry, exhibit, and wildlife raptors are reviewed with regard to factors that affect their mortality, life expectancy, and age evaluation. In addition, medical conditions that are frequently seen in geriatric raptors are covered in this article.

species with continually growing (elodont) teeth. This feature allows the geriatric rabbit to possess teeth that are essentially "new", a distinct advantage over geriatric carnivores. Expanded longevity, while generally desirable, necessarily accompanies an increase in geriatric disorders. This article examines the spectrum of disease that can affect the geriatric rabbit as well as crucial factors concerning the clinical management of the animal up to the end of its life. An improved understanding of geriatric disorders in pet rabbits allows early recognition and the opportunity to improve quality of life.

Aging processes leading to specific organ problems are not obvious in aging psittacines. In general, birds live long and age slowly despite their high metabolic rates and very high total lifetime energy expenditures. Most pathologic processes seen in older parrots are generally not specific for aging because they are seen in young birds as well. Pathologic processes that have a tendency to occur more in older psittacines are atherosclerosis and repeated injury processes, such as chronic pulmonary interstitial fibrosis, pneumoconiosis, liver fibrosis, and lens cataracts. Also, some neoplasms are more often seen at an older age.

I would like to especially thank Dr Patricia Gray, our avian resident and my co-guest editor, who spent long hours assisting me in the editorial process.

I hope this issue helps to spur further interest in the area of geriatric avian and exotic medicine.

Sharman M. Hoppes, DVM, DABVP-Avian
Department of Veterinary Small Animal Clinical Sciences
College of Veterinary Medicine and Biomedical Sciences
Texas A&M University, 4474 TAMU
College Station, TX 77843-4474, USA

E-mail address:
Shoppes@cvm.tamu.edu (S.M. Hoppes)

In this issue of *Veterinary Clinics of North America: Exotic Animal Practice*, the focus is on the medical care of elderly exotic patients. It is not surprising that this is the first such issue since the periodical's inception in 1998. There has not been a whole lot published regarding the aged exotic patient. The focus has been on exotic animal husbandry and medicine in general, and with good reason. As is the case for more conventional companion animals, our care of exotic pets has improved dramatically over the past few decades, and our patients are actually living long enough to develop purely age-related health problems.

My two senior cats (Porcupine and Lizzy) both passed away recently. Watching them slow down with age over the past couple of years was hard for my husband and me. We knew they were starting to feel the effects of time, and that they would not be with us much longer. What helped us (and them) through this process was our awareness level as far as what to expect and how we could manage them as geriatric patients. The knowledge that we were doing everything medically possible to keep them comfortable and happy was very empowering, and when they did finally leave us we were able to say with certainty that they'd had a terrific life—from start to finish.

Every one of our patients deserves the best medical care we have to offer, on all levels. Aging brings about disease processes that can be very challenging, both to owners and to veterinarians. To provide the kind of preventive and palliative care necessary when dealing with our geriatric patients, we need to know what to expect. Although certain processes appear to be universal across species, we need to be aware of the many species-specific peculiarities with regard to aging. The following articles were compiled by veterinarians well versed in the care of elderly exotic animals, and I hope readers will take advantage of the information shared here when dealing with their senior patients.

I would like to thank Sharman Hoppes for inviting me to work on this project with her. It's been a very rewarding experience. I would also like to thank the contributing authors for their hard work: It is much appreciated.

This issue is dedicated to beloved elderly pets everywhere, be they 3-year-old rats, 33-year-old chinchillas, 55-year-old parrots, or 99-year-old fish.

Patricia Gray, DVM, MS
Zoological Medicine/Schubot Exotic Bird Health Center
College of Veterinary Medicine and Biomedical Sciences
Texas A&M University
College Station, TX 77843-4474, USA

E-mail address:
Pgray@cvm.tamu.edu (P. Gray)

Geriatric Veterinary Care for Fish Patients

E. Scott Weber III, VMD, MSc Aquatic Vet Sci/Pathobiology

KEYWORDS
- Fish longevity • Environmental quality • Infectious disease
- Fish reproduction

There is little evidence-based research and scientific literature available for providing geriatric care for fish patients. Fish can have tremendous longevity. Although the average life span for most fish species can be only a few days to weeks for the beginning hobbyist, it is becoming more common for clients to have animals for several decades with the advent and continued development of improved life-support systems, husbandry, water quality additives, and fish nutrition. This article discusses fish longevity for several popular species, addresses environmental quality issues for geriatric patients, and provides information on the most common challenges, from a veterinary perspective, to maintain fish over the years.

FISH LONGEVITY AND SENESCENCE

Several commonly kept species of fish have life spans that rival and greatly exceed many other vertebrates kept as domestic pets. As recently as the 1970s, a few academicians theorized that fish were unique in that they do not age, but others have published literature reviews and research from senescence studies in guppies refuting this hypothesis.[1] Some researchers have shown longevity increases with genome size in Acipenseriformes, Cypriniformes, and Salmoniformes.[2] Because fish are highly represented with a large number of species known to live for more than 100 years, work by Reznick and colleagues[3] suggests that, unlike birds and mammals, fish have evolved delayed senescence based on increased fecundity with age, that slower growth delays maturity, and that lower mortality rates lead to maximum life spans similar to birds and mammals. Guppies have been used as a model for understanding evolutionary theory and natural senescence, linking age-specific changes in reproduction with mortality rates, and showing that reproductively active animals may age more quickly.[4,5] Other factors may also play a part in aging of captive and wild fish species including water temperature, marine verses freshwater environs, and deep dwelling

Aquatic Animal Health, VM: Medicine and Epidemiology, University of California, Davis, 2108 Tupper Hall, Davis, CA 95616, USA
E-mail address: epweber@ucdavis.edu

Vet Clin Exot Anim 13 (2010) 1–14
doi:10.1016/j.cvex.2009.11.001
1094-9194/10/$ – see front matter © 2010 Elsevier Inc. All rights reserved.

Table 1
Commonly kept fish species and record life spans

Order/Family	Genus/Species	Common Name	Wild (Y)	Captivity	References
Poeciliidae	*Gambusia affinis*	Mosquito fish, gambusia	1.5	—	Altman & Dittmer[9]; Krumholtz[10]
Cyprinidae	*Barbus bynni bynni*	Niger barb (+)	—	16.3	Altman & Dittmer[9]; Flower[11]
	Carassius auratus	Goldfish	41.0	30.0	Flower[11]; Carlander[12]; Moyle[13]; Bobick & Peffer[14]
	Cyprinius carpio	Carp	38.0	47.0	Flower[15], Hinton[16]
	Cyprinus carassius auratus	Goldfish/carp hybrid	—	10.0	Flower[11]
	Leuciscus orfus	Golden orfe (+)	—	14.25	Flower[11]
Syngnathidae	*Hippocampus hippocampus*	Short-snouted sea horse	—	1.3	Altman & Dittmer[9]; Flower[11]
	Hippocampus erectus	Atlantic-lined sea horse or Northern sea horse	1.0	—	Herald & Rakowicz[17]; Strawn[18]
Mormyridae	*Gnathonemus cyprinoides*	Trunkfish	—	7.1	Flower[11]
	Pollimyrus isidori isidori	Mormyrid (+)	29	28.0	Altman & Dittmer[9]; Flower[15]; Hinton[16]
	Mormyrus kannume	Elephant-snout fish (+)	—	6.3	Flower[11]
Notopteridae	*Xenomystus nigri*	African brown knifefish	—	11.4	Altman & Dittmer[9]; Flower[11]
Osteoglossidae	*Osteoglossum bicirrhosum*	South American silver arowana	6.5	—	Hinton[16]
Anabantidae	*Ctenopoma kingsleyae*	Tail-spot climbing perch	—	8.7	Altman & Dittmer[9]; Flower[11]
	Anabas testudineus	Climbing perch	—	11.0	Altman & Dittmer[9]; Flower[15]
	Macropodus opercularis	Paradise fish	—	8.0	Altman & Dittmer[9]; Flower[11]
Chaetodontidae	*Chaetodon lineolatus*	Lined butterflyfish	10.0	—	Hinton[16]
	Chaetodon lunula	Raccoon butterflyfish	9.0	—	Hinton[16]
	Chelmon rostratus	Copperband butterflyfish	10.0	—	Hinton[16]
	Forcipiger flavissimus	Long-nosed butterflyfish	18.0	—	Hinton[16]
Cichlidae	*Acara tetramerus*	Two-spot acara, saddle cichlid	—	7.0	Altman & Dittmer[9]; Flower[11]
	Cichlasoma cyanoguttatum	Rio Grande perch, Texas cichlid	—	5.0	Altman & Dittmer[9]; Flower[15]
	Tilapia spp	African cichlid	—	7.0	Altman & Dittmer[9]; Flower[11]
Labridae	*Coris julis*	Mediterranean rainbow wrasse	7.0	—	Hinton[16]

Family	Species	Common name			Reference
Pomacanthidae	Centropyge flavissimus	Lemonpeel angelfish	11.0	—	Hinton[16]
	Euxiphipops navarchus	Blue-girdled angelfish	15.0	—	Hinton[16]
	Pomacanthus imperator	Emperor angelfish	14.0	—	Hinton[16]
	Pygoplites diacanthus	Regal angelfish	14.5	—	Hinton[16]
	Amphiprion clarkia	Clarkii clownfish, Clark's anemonefish	11.0	—	Moyer[19]
	Amphiprion ephippium	Fire clownfish	16.0	—	Hinton[16]
	Dascyllus aruanus	Three-stripe damsel, Humbug dascyllus, Banded dascyllus	6.0	—	Hinton[16]
	Centropyge tibicen	Keyhole angelfish	6.0	—	Moyer[19]
Polypteridae	Polypterus senegalus	Cuvier's bichir	—	34.0	Altman & Dittmer[9]; Flower[15]
Clariidae	Clarias lazera	African walking catfish (+)	—	16.2	Altman & Dittmer[9]; Flower[11]
Ictaluridae	Ictalurus lacustris punctatus	Albino channel catfish	13.0	—	Altman & Dittmer[9]; Lewis[20]
Loricariidae	Hypostomus punctatus	Common plecostomus	18.0	—	Hinton[16]
Mochokidae	Synodontis schall	Upside-down catfish	12.0	31.0	Flower[11]; Hinton[16]
Pimelodidae	Pimelodus spp	Pim catfish	—	7.0	Altman & Dittmer[9]; Flower[11]
Tetraodontidae	Canthigaster solandri	Common sharpnose puffer	7.0	—	Altman & Dittmer[9]; Flower[15]

+ indicates that individual was still alive at the time that life span was recorded.

Data from Carey JR, Judge DS. Longevity records: life spans of mammals, birds, amphibians, reptiles, and fish. Monographs on population aging, 8. Rostock (Germany): Odense University Press, Max-Planck-Geselschaft; 2002. Available at: http://www.demogr.mpg.de/?http://www.demogr.mpg.de/longevityrecords/.

This disease was first reported in 1897 by Bataillon in a common carp, and the three most commonly recognized etiologic agents of atypical mycobacteriosis in fish are *Mycobacterium marinum, Mycobacterium fortuitum, and Mycobacterium chelonae* in ornamental fish.[41]

Clinical signs of mycobacteriosis include listlessness, lethargy, and isolation from other fish.[42] Many animals may exhibit emaciation, dermatitis, exophthalmia, ascites, coelomic distension, or ulceration. Fish can exhibit profound emaciation despite a voracious appetite, and some fish have extensive epaxial-muscle wasting making them resemble a tadpole or lollipop. Many animals have skin ulcerations that may or may not have skeletal-muscle involvement, and in a few cases spinal lesions have been documented causing scoliosis and lytic changes in the bone.[42] Fish may be infected, with or without clinical signs, from weeks to years. Gross necropsy lesions caused by mycobacteriosis include gray/white to tan miliary granulomas found in virtually any parenchymatous tissue; the spleen, kidney, and liver are the most common organs affected.[42] Enlarged organs, coelomitis, and coelomic fluid may be apparent. Transmission of this bacterium is primarily through consumption of contaminated feed, cannibalism of infected fish, or aquatic detritus. Environmental conditions including low levels of dissolved oxygen, low pH, high organic loads, and warm water predispose to infectious outbreaks.

There is no ante mortem testing available for diagnosing atypical mycobacteriosis in fish patients. Acid-fast staining of anal swabs can give misleading results and lead to diagnosing false-positive animals in infected systems because of the ubiquitous nature of the pathogen, the possibility of mycobacteria passing through the fish's gastrointestinal tract, and the presence of other acid-fast staining bacteria.[43] A negative result may simply suggest an animal is not shedding mycobacteria at the time of testing. Histopathology with Fite's acid-fast stain is the current method of choice when coupled with molecular diagnostics and clinical symptoms. Polymerase chain reaction of infected tissues as a confirmatory test is sensitive and accurate and offers rapid results, but is also expensive. Culture of affected tissues coupled with molecular testing and histopathology is the gold standard, but it can take several months to finalize results, which makes this impractical in more acute outbreaks.

There is currently no effective treatment for mycobacteriosis, although several experimental regimens have been tried.[44] Treatment suggestions that are reported have not all been supported with histopathology to determine if infections were truly cleared, and many treatment recommendations fell far short of time intervals required to treat other atypical mycobacterial pathogens in terrestrial animals.[45] Another caveat with treatment is the antibiotic treatment regimens and treatment duration for mycobacteriosis in an aquarium or pond, lends to potential antibiotic misuse and bacterial resistance. Management is the only method for controlling this disease until sensitive, specific, expedient, and affordable antemortem testing and treatments become available. Management varies from conservative approaches of zero tolerance for suspected cases with euthanasia and disinfection of systems, to ignoring the pathogen entirely with no action for clinically suspect animals.

Atypical mycobacteriosis can cause infections in humans and other mammals. Tuberculoid infections in humans using public swimming pools were first reported in 1939 in Sweden and cases in the United States emerged in 1951. The causative organism, *Mycobacterium marinum,* was identified in 1954 and is referred to today as "fish tank granuloma."[46] All fish should be handled as if they may contain mycobacteria and people who have cuts on their hands or those who are immunocompromised for any reason are at greatest risk.

REPRODUCTIVE PROBLEMS

Many species of fish do not readily breed in captivity. Because of environmental threats and decreasing habitat, breeding fish in captivity may become necessary for the survival of several species in the wild. Fish reproductive problems and anomalies are a common occurrence in public and home aquaria. In the past, many of these cases were diagnosed on necropsy. With advances in fish medicine, reproductive problems are being diagnosed antemortem to allow for treatments. Diagnosis of reproductive related disease begins with a thorough history and water quality evaluation, and knowledge of the individual species' reproductive physiology. Some diagnostic modalities that can be used to evaluate the fish patient are complete blood counts, blood chemistries, ultrasound, radiology with/without contrast, computer assisted tomography, general palpation, laparoscopy, cystocentesis, and cloacal endoscopy.[47] The most common problems encountered clinically include dystocia or egg binding, cystic ovaries, infectious disease, organ prolapse, organ trauma, secondary bacterial infections, and neoplasia. Specific treatments for reproductive problems in fish can include hormonal treatment, surgery, antibiotic or antifungal therapy, environmental changes, and improved nutrition.

NEOPLASIA

Fish are regularly used in environmental and chemical testing to detect and study effects of mutagenic pollutants or compounds.[48] Similar to other vertebrates, several different tumors have been isolated and identified in fish. Many of these tumors have been recorded and archived at the George Washington University Medical Center Registry of Tumors in Lower Animals. Although the significance of tumorigenesis in fish has been primarily of a scientific nature, in the last decade veterinarians have begun diagnosing and treating cancers in a variety of teleosts. Several diagnostic and treatment options have been used for treatment of fish. Weisse and colleagues[49] described the successful removal of a seminoma in a black sea bass (*Centropristis striata*), diagnosing the animal using contrast radiography, contrast spiral CT, and ultrasonography. Harms and colleagues used microsurgery for the removal of an abdominal mass in a gourami, and Lewbart and colleagues also performed surgery to treat an undifferentiated abdominal sarcoma in a koi (*C carpio*).[50,51] Neoplastic lesions can occur anywhere, and in goldfish (*Carassius auratas*) a dermal fibrosarcoma has been reported.[52] Other unpublished cases include diagnosis of intracoelomic lipomas using advanced imaging in goldfish (*C auratas*); koi (*C carpio*); catfish (*Synodontis* sp); and largemouth bass (*Micropterus salmoides*) by the author and Dr Tobias Schwartz at the University of Edinburgh; cryosurgical intervention for squamous cell carcinoma in a kannume (*Mormyrus kannume*) over 6 months managed by Drs Lance Adams, Leslie Boerner, and the author at the New England Aquarium; lymphosarcoma diagnosed in brook trout (*Salvelinus fontinalis*) by the author and Dr Charles Innis at the New England Aquarium; and radiation, surgical, and cryosurgical intervention for a neurofibroma of a goldfish (*C auratas*) performed at Tufts under direction of Dr Joerg Mayer. Diagnostics for neoplasia cases include survey radiography, ultrasonography, positive-contrast radiography, hematology, blood-chemistry analysis, histopathology, and CT. One of the greatest challenges for aquatic animal veterinarians is getting an early and quick diagnosis. In the absence of other clinical abnormalities or behavioral changes, abdominal masses are difficult to detect until abdominal distension is observed. Often, when abdominal distension is first observed, tumors have grown substantially in size and may account for up to 25% or more of the animal's body weight. Other types of cancer, such as

12. Carlander KD. Handbook of freshwater biology I. In: Life history data on freshwater fishes of the United States and Canada, exclusive of the perciformes, vol. 1. Ames (IA): Iowa State University Press; 1969.

13. Moyle PB. Inland fishes of California. Berkeley (CA): University California Press; 1976.

14. Bobick JE, Peffer M, editors. Science and technology desk reference. Washington, DC: Gale Research Inc; 1993.

15. Flower MSS. Further notes on the duration of life in animals. - I. Fishes: as determined by otolith and scale - readings and direct observations on living animals. Proc Zool Soc Lond 1935;(2):265–304.

16. Hinton. Horned shark, gar, mormyriad, characin, carp, armored catfish, arowana, upside down catfish. Available at: http://www.demogr.mpg.de/?http://www.demogr.mpg.de/longevityrecords/.

17. Herald ES, Rakowicz M. Stable requirements for raising sea horses. Aquarium J 1951;22:234–42.

18. Strawn K. Life history of the pygmy seahorse, *Hippocampus zosterae* (Jordan and Gilbert) at Cedar Key, Florida. Copeia 1958;16–22.

19. Moyer JT. Longevity of the anemone fish *Amphiprion clarkii* at Miyake-jima, Japan with notes on four other species. Copeia 1986;1:135–9.

20. Lewis WM. Fisheries investigations on two artificial lakes in southern Iowa II. Fish populations. Iowa State Coll J Sci 1950;24:287.

21. Lewis WM, Morris DP. Toxicity of nitrite: a review. Trans Am Fish Soc 1986;115: 183–95.

22. Camargo JA, Alonso A, Salamanca A. Nitrate toxicity to aquatic animals: a review with new data for freshwater invertebrates. Chemosphere 2005;58:1255–67.

23. Hamlin HJ. Nitrate toxicity in Siberian sturgeon (*Acipenser baeri*). Aquaculture 2006;253:688–93.

24. Shaw BJ, Handy RD. Dietary copper exposure and recovery in Nile tilapia, *Oreochromis niloticus*. Aquat Toxicol 2006;76:111–21.

25. Carrola J, Fontaínhas-Fernandes A, Rocha M. Liver histopathology in brown trout (*Salmo trutta f. fario*) from the Tinhela river, subjected to mine drainage from the abandoned Jales mine (Portugal). Bull Environ Contam Toxicol 2009;83:35–41.

26. Wolf JC, Wolfe MJ. A brief overview of nonneoplastic hepatic toxicity in fish. Toxicol Pathol 2005;33:75–85.

27. Weber E Scott, Newman M. Hydrogen sulfide as a cause of mortality in baitfish ponds. Arkansas Aquafarming 2000;17(1):3–5.

28. Brown SB, Honeyfield DC, Vandenbyllaardt L. Thiamine analysis in fish tissues. Am Fish Soc Symp 1998;21:73–81.

29. Jaroszewska M, Lee B-J, Dabrowski K, et al. Effects of vitamin B1 (thiamine) deficiency in lake trout (*Salvelinus namaycush*) alevins at hatching stage. Comp Biochem Physiol A Mol Integr Physiol 2009;154:255–62.

30. Koski P, Soivio A, Hartikainen K, et al. M74 syndrome and thiamine in salmon broodfish and offspring. Boreal Env Res 2001;6:79–92.

31. Tillitt DE, Zajicek JL, Brown SB, et al. Thiamine and thiaminase status in forage fish of salmonines from Lake Michigan. J Aquat Anim Health 2005;17:13–25.

32. Crow GL, Luer WH, Harshbarger JC, et al. Relationship of water chemistry to serum thyroid hormones in captive sharks with goiters. Aquat Geochem 1998; 4:469–80.

33. Sonstegard R, Leatherland JF. The epizootiology and pathogenesis of thyroid hyperplasia in coho salmon (*Oncorhynchus kisutch*) in Lake Ontario. Cancer Res 1976;36:4467–75.

34. Crow GL, Luer WH, Harshbarger JC. Histological assessment of goiters in elasmobranch fishes. J Aquat Anim Health 2001;13:1–7.
35. Nigrelli RF, Ruggieri GD. Hyperplasia and neoplasia of the thyroid in marine fishes. Mt Sinai J Med 1973;41:283–93.
36. El-Zayadi Abdel-Rahman. Hepatic steatosis: a benign disease or a silent killer. World J Gastroenterol 2008;14(26):4120–6.
37. Spisni E, Tugnoli M, Ponticelli A, et al. Hepatic steatosis in artificially fed marine teleosts. J Fish Dis 1998;21:177–84.
38. Henderson RJ. Fatty acid metabolism in freshwater fish with particular reference to polyunsaturated fatty acids. Arch Tierernahr 1996;49:5–22.
39. Yılmaz E, Genc E. Effects of alternative dietary lipid sources (Soy-acid oil and Yellow grease) on growth and hepatic lipidosis of common carp (*Cyprinus carpio*) fingerling: a preliminary study. Turk J Fish Aquat Sci 2006;6:37–42.
40. Montero D, Robaina LE, Socorro J, et al. Alteration of liver and muscle fatty acid composition in gilthead sea bream (*Sparus aurata*) juveniles held at high stocking density and fed an essential fatty acid deficient diet. Fish Physiol Biochem 2001; 24:63–72.
41. Gauthier DT, Rhodes MW. Mycobacteriosis in fishes: a review. Vet J 2009;180(1):5–6.
42. Roberts H, Palmiero B, Weber ES. Bacterial and parasitic diseases of fish. Vet Clin North Am Exot Anim Pract 2009;12(3):609–38.
43. Weber ES. Gastroenterology for the piscine patient. Vet Clin North Am Exot Anim Pract 2005;8:247–76.
44. Boos S, Schmidt H, Ritter G, et al. Effectiveness of oral rifampicin against myco-bacteriosis in tropical fish. Berl Munch Tierarztl Wochenschr 1995;108(7):253–5.
45. Conroy G, Conroy DA. Acid-fast bacterial infection and its control in guppies (*Lebistes reticulatus*) reared on an ornamental fish farm in Venezuela. Vet Rec 1999;144:177–8.
46. Decostere A, Hermans K, Haesebrouck F. Piscine mycobacteriosis: a literature review covering the agent and the disease it causes in fish and humans. Vet Microbiol 2004;99(3–4):159–66.
47. Weber ES 3rd, Weisse C, Schwarz T, et al. Anesthesia, diagnostic imaging, and surgery of fish. Compend Contin Educ Vet 2009;31(2):E1–9 [online].
48. Groff JM. Neoplasia in fishes. Vet Clin North Am Exot Anim Pract 2004;7(3): 705–56.
49. Weisse C, Weber ES, Matzkin Z, et al. Surgical removal of a seminoma from a Black Sea Bass (*Centropristis striata*). J Am Vet Med Assoc 2002;220(2):280–3.
50. Harms CA, Bakal RS, Khoo LH, et al. Microsurgical excision of an abdominal mass in a gourami. J Am Vet Med Assoc 1995;207:1215–7.
51. Lewbart GA, Spodnick G, Barlow N, et al. Surgical removal of an undifferentiated abdominal sarcoma from a koi carp (*Cyprinus carpio*). Vet Rec 1998;143:556–8.
52. Probasco D, Noga EJ, Marcellin D, et al. Dermal fibrosarcoma in a goldfish; case report. J Small Exotic Anim Med 1994;2:173–5.
53. Harms CA, Lewbart GA. Surgery in fish. In: Bennett RA, editor. Vet Clin North Am Exotic Anim Pract 2000;3:759–74.
54. Scientific American PBS Broadcast. Available at: http://www.pbs.org/saf/transcripts/transcript805.htm. Accessed August 1, 2009.
55. Ashton N, Brown N, Easty D. Trematode cataract in fresh water fish. J Small Anim Pract 1969;10:471–8.
56. Bjerka E, Bjerka I, Moksness E. An outbreak of cataract with lens rupture and nuclear extrusion in wolf-fish (*Anarhicas* spp). Vet Ophthalmol 1998;1(1):9–15.

age-related increases in mortality, decreased reproduction, and general physical deterioration revealed in various pathologies.[6] Ageing in reptiles was previously reviewed in 1976[7] and later in 1994.[8,9] Little more data have come to light since. Three types of senescence are known to occur in reptiles.[8,9] Most squamates studied to date seem to undergo gradual senescence after maturity, similar to mammals and birds. In chelonians and crocodilians, growth continues throughout life and senescence is imperceptible or negligible. At the other end of the spectrum, rapid senescence and death following sexual maturity and mating, similar to that seen in salmon and small dasyurid marsupials, occurs in a few small reptiles and is best documented in Buettner's mabuya, *Mabuya* (*Trachylepis*) *buettneri*, a small African skink. Actual measurement of senescence can be achieved in several ways, and those methods are reviewed by Patnaik.[8] At the population level, an increase in the mortality rate would be expected with senescence, yet that is not always the case in reptiles studied to date.[8] At the individual level, experimental measurements of quantifiable age-related changes in metabolic function parameters, such as tissue glucose uptake, muscular glycolysis, tricarboxylic acid (TCA [Krebs]) cycle, cell membrane cholesterol/phospholipid ratio, hepatic antioxidant level, brain antioxidative enzymes, collagen cross-linkage, and enzyme thermolability, have been used to assess rates and patterns of senescence in various species of reptiles,[8] but such tests are not practical and are of little value in a clinical setting. This is unfortunate as reptiles are remarkable at concealing their age (**Fig. 1**). External features or lesions suggestive of old age in reptiles may be more a function of prior disease or trauma or may reflect inadequate or substandard husbandry (**Fig. 2**).

AGE ESTIMATION IN REPTILES

The determination of longevity and expected lifespan in a given species relies on data collected from specimens of known or estimated age. Techniques used in age determination of reptiles were reviewed by Castanet.[10] Prospective studies are lacking in cohorts of reptiles for which an accurate or close estimate of the hatching/birth date is known. Ironically, the long lifespan of many reptiles somewhat impedes or prohibits such studies. As juvenile captive-bred reptiles become increasingly popular in the pet trade, longevity in these species is likely to become better defined. However, owners or caregivers are typically unaware of the age of their pet reptile, and reptiles

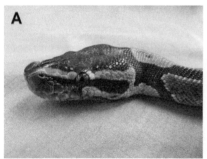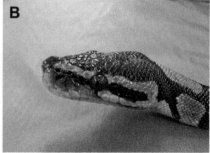

Fig. 1. Head of a 12-year-old (*A*) and a 40-year-old (*B*) ball python. The scales on the head of the older python are mildly raised and the epidermis between the scales is visible, imparting a slightly rougher outline to the skin; this could be an individual variation rather than one due to age. Estimating the age of a snake based on geriatric physical changes is difficult-to-impossible.

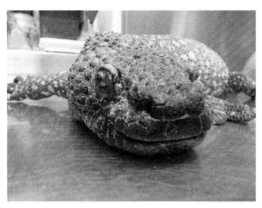

Fig. 2. Head of a 41-year-old Mexican beaded lizard (*Heloderma horridum horridum*). Bilateral idiopathic buphthalmia and slight bulging of the third eyelid has been present for over a decade, and has required periodic medical management.

show few, if any, outward signs of ageing. Although desirable, there is no useful noninvasive method for the clinician or caregiver to assess the age of a given individual reptile. Even size is not always reliable. Growth in most reptiles occurs throughout life[11] and although body size is positively correlated with age, even morphometric criteria or growth curves/charts established for wild individuals may be skewed in captivity as growth can be significantly affected by feeding regimen and husbandry. Deficiencies lead to stunting whereas overfeeding, or power-feeding, accelerates growth. Size can therefore be misleading, yet it may remain the best clue in younger animals of many species. Field biologists rely on the mark-release-recapture technique to assess longevity and other demographic patterns in wild reptiles.[11] Sclerochronology and skeletochronology refer to age estimation using natural growth marks in epidermal scutes and bone, respectively. The latter involves reading thin histologic bone sections and is more precise but clinically impractical because bones could hardly be harvested from the living pet; sclerochronology, or scute ring measurement, is less accurate and relies on growth cycles that may or may not be annual, especially for captive reptiles housed in an artificial, controlled environment (**Fig. 3**).[11] Furthermore, scutes in individual animals may be subject to uneven or excessive wear. Nevertheless, papers describing the use of sclerochronology in more than 20 chelonian species are listed in Castanet, 1994[11] and could be used to estimate the age of captive chelonians. Wilson and colleagues,[12] in 2003, provided a synopsis of the anatomy and physiology of growth ring deposition and critically reviewed prior sclerochronological studies in chelonians. Rattlesnakes (genera *Crotalus* and *Sistrurus*) add a segment to their rattle with each ecdysis so that a crude age may be estimated by counting segments, but shedding in snakes is irregular, may occur 2 to 3 times each year, and the rattle often breaks as it gains in length. Other methods of age assessment, such as measurement of telomere length in erythrocytes,[13] may show some potential in the future because it could be estimated from a simple blood sample.

LONGEVITY IN REPTILES

A geriatric reptile is one approaching the end of its lifespan. Owners often ask clinicians how long their pet will live. An awareness of the expected lifespan of a reptile

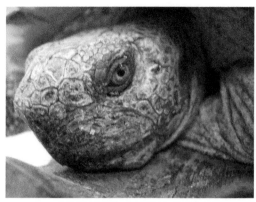

Fig. 4. Head of a 100-years-old desert tortoise. There is slight hyperkeratosis over the scales of the head. (*Courtesy of* Jeri Oliphant, DVM, Arcata, CA).

Bearded dragons live 8 to 10 years,[17] possibly up to 14, and have a relatively short lifespan by reptilian standards. Other common captive agamids, such as the green water dragon (*Physignathus cocincinus*) and uromastyx lizards (*Uromastyx* spp) may live slightly longer. Green iguanas (*Iguana iguana*) typically live 10 to 15 years, but some have lived more than 20 years. Anoles (*Anolis* sp), commonly sold in pet shops, live 5 to 7 years. Leopard geckos have been known to live between 20 and 30 years, and that may be true of other eublepharine lizards, such as the African fat-tailed gecko (*Hemitheconyx caudicinctus*). A shorter lifespan of 10 to 15 years is reported for day geckos (*Phelsuma* spp) and New Caledonian crested geckos. Blue-tongued skinks (*Tiliqua scincoides*) and tegus (*Tupinambis* spp) have a life expectancy of 15 to 20 years. Life expectancy may be slightly less for savannah monitors (*Varanus exanthematicus*). Readers are referred to Slavens and Slavens,[17] 2009 for species not listed here. As more information becomes available and better care is provided to pet and captive reptiles, life expectancy may be extended.

CLINICAL CONSIDERATIONS

The authors propose that geriatric care of captive reptiles starts with the first consultation. Thorough questioning of the caregiver allows for a critical review of husbandry and provision of sound advice, which in turn, hopefully translates into an extended captive lifespan. Owners should be warned that reptiles are stoic animals and that they exhibit a very limited range of clinical signs. The onset of age-related ailments may be insidious and can be preceded by subtle decline in performance and vigor. In addition to monitoring appetite and fecal/urinary output, caregivers should be instructed to objectively and critically examine their animal regularly. A precision scale should be used to weigh their reptile weekly, or at least monthly, and weight entered into a log so that any trend might be detected. Weight loss, which can be gradual and easily go unnoticed, is often the first sign of a problem. Captive reptiles should ideally undergo a complete veterinary physical examination yearly. The oral cavity, nares, eyes, ears, integument, vent, feet and nails, and tail should be carefully inspected. Cardiac auscultation is typically unrewarding in reptiles, and palpation is limited in chelonians and somewhat restricted in many lizards and snakes, all reasons why ancillary tests are particularly useful in assessing health. Serial blood sampling and imaging, initiated at maturity or earlier, are undoubtedly the most powerful tools for the diagnosis, monitoring, and management of geriatric issues. Although criteria for normality are fairly well established in cats and dogs, the same is not true for reptiles, which is why blood parameters and radiographs are best compared with blood results and radiographs taken earlier in life for each individual. In most reptile species, blood collection and radiographic imaging are fairly straightforward and do not require sedation or immobilization. Successive blood work and radiographs establish baselines for each individual reptile and can be repeated every second year, yearly, or even more often, as the patient ages. Serial blood work provides a better grasp of normal seasonal or physiologic fluctuation in blood parameter values in a given individual and allows the clinician to detect trends even when reference ranges for the species are unavailable (**Table 1**). Such trends may provide the clinician with grounds for focused individual geriatric care targeting a specific organ system and an objective means of assessing efficacy of therapeutic or supportive measures. Anemia, infection, parasitemia, hepatic and renal function, hypercholesterolemia, calcium homeostasis, and glycemia are among conditions for which blood parameters may change over the years. Yearly radiographs optimize the odds of detecting bone and soft tissue changes in an individual reptile (**Fig. 5**). Degenerative joint disease, spondylopathy, atherosclerosis, dystrophic mineralization, uroliths, cardiomegaly, hepatomegaly, renomegaly, coelomic masses, folliculogenesis, gravidity, pneumonia, and foreign bodies are among conditions that may be diagnosed radiographically. Most may

Table 1
Serial blood sample values of a female ornate Nile monitor lizard (*Varanus ornatus*) over the years. Individual variations in blood parameters are appreciable and allow for better interpretation of blood results should the animal become sick

Date	2001-07-01	2004-01-05	2006-01-06	2008-01-08
Hematology				
PCV (%)	37	32	21	27
RBC (10^6/μL)	0.7	1.0	0.8	0.8
Hb (g/L)	173	124	113	128
WBC (10^3/μL)	0.36	3.33	1.54	2.82
%Heterophils	79	50	34	47
%Lymphocytes	01	29	51	16
%Monocytes	—	6	—	3
%Azurophils	18	15	15	16
%Eosinophils	—	—	—	—
%Basophils	2	—	—	1
Chemistry				
Total protein (g/L)	36	68	47	51
Glucose (mmol/L)	2.2	8.8	5.4	3.5
Uric acid (μmol/L)	76	723	485	91
Calcium (mmol/L)	NA	10.72	2.81	8.67
Phosph (mmol/L)	NA	2.52	1.44	2.95
CK (IU/L)	NA	231	1286	1097
AST (IU/L)	NA	14	30	19

Abbreviations: AST, aspartate aminotransferase; CK, creatine kinase; Hb, hemoglohin; PCV, packed cell volume; Phosph, phosphorus; RBC, red blood cell; WBC, white blood cell.

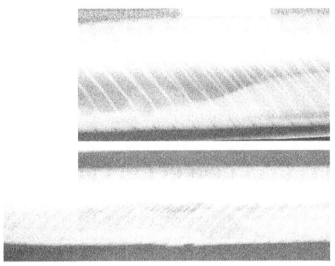

Fig. 5. Lateral plain radiographic view of the caudal lung field of a male tiger rat snake (*Spilotes pullatus*) at age 5 (*A*) and 6 (*B*) years. Hyperostotic spondylopathy is slightly more pronounced and the aorta is more radiodense at age 6 years.

easily be subclinical and not be identified on physical examination. As in most vertebrate species, neoplasia in all organ systems is seen with increased frequency in older reptiles. When diagnosed early, some of these conditions may be addressed therapeutically or may be decelerated by means of dietary or husbandry recommendations, increasing the life expectancy of the patient. Additional diagnostic modalities, such as magnetic resonance imaging, bone scans, and endoscopy require immobilization and are now available to further define lesions or assess progression of disease in the older patient. Anesthesia in older reptiles, as in other geriatric vertebrates, might come with an increased risk of complications. The newer volatile anesthetics combined with short-acting or reversible drug combinations probably offer the widest safety margins. Tracheal intubation, placement of an intravenous or intraosseous access line, and the use of monitoring devices will help detect a complication and allow for early intervention. With careful planning, the need for anesthesia should not deter the clinician, owner, or caregiver from pursuing advanced diagnostics for captive reptiles.

The following list is by no means exhaustive, but includes the most common conditions associated with ageing in reptiles.

Integument

Skin lesions are most easily noticed by caregivers. Scars are common in older reptiles. Skin tone and gloss may or may not be decreased. Ecdysis may be less frequent in older squamates but may also be more frequent with age or disease. Hyperkeratosis, cutaneous growths and excrescences, broken tails and regrowths, missing toes and/ or nails, and overgrown beaks are more common in aged animals.

Digestive System

Anorexia is probably the **most common clinical sign displayed by sick or geriatric** reptiles, but is very nonspecific. Periodontal disease is seen in older lizards, especially in acrodont species (eg, Agamidae, Chamaeleonidae). Delayed gastrointestinal transit

een in older
prevalent in
snakes, so
benefit from
nd judicious

lea, bradyp-
rea, and dyspn   pulmonary disease or   or metabolic
disturbances. O   eathing is typically ass   ous tracheal
or lung pathology.

Cardiovascular System

Atherosclerosis and dystrophic myocardial mineralization are common in older snakes and lizards. Death may be peracute when an affected artery ruptures. Luminal narrowing of aortic arches, carotids, and cerebral vessels may lead to more subtle and progressive signs, neurologic or other. Hypercholesteremia is often seen, and the causes are poorly understood. The use of cholesterol-lowering drugs in such animals remains unexplored.

Urinary System

Chronic, progressive renal disease is fairly common in older squamates. In many lizards, nephrosis and renal swelling may impinge on the colon at the pelvic inlet, which commonly results in constipation, particularly in green iguanas. Secondary renal hyperparathyroidism is sometimes seen, as serum calcium levels drop and phosphorus levels rise. Articular gout causes painful swelling of the limbs. Visceral gout, insidious and difficult to diagnose, may cause death with no premonitory signs or may cause various degrees of lethargy, anorexia, and other nonspecific signs. The efficacy and safety of allopurinol, colchicine, and other drugs targeting the uric acid pathway are largely unknown. Fluid therapy and diuresis, dietary adjustments, and pain management are more likely to help hyperuricemic reptiles. Renal neoplasia occurs in all reptiles, but seems unusually prevalent in older kingsnakes and milksnakes (*Lampropeltis* spp).

Reproductive System

Reptiles typically remain reproductively active throughout their life. Reproductive senility, as measured by decreased reproductive output, occurs in most vertebrates but is poorly documented in reptiles. Although a reproductive decline with old age has been documented in some crocodilians, oogonial proliferation is known to persist late into adulthood of at least some alligators (*A mississippiensis*) and clutch size seems to increase with age in some snakes, lizards, and turtles.[8] Older female reptiles may be more at risk of follicular stasis or dystocia, because they may be obese or more likely to be struggling with calcium homeostasis. Yolk coelomitis and ovarian neoplasia sometimes occur. Infection or impaction of the hemipenal pockets in lizards and snakes tend to be seen more often in older individuals.

Nervous System

Neurologic signs in reptiles include incoordination or ataxia, opisthotonos or star-gazing, loss of righting reflex, tremors, and seizures. Tremors and fasciculations in old reptiles are almost always related to hypocalcemia and are not truly neurologic. Brain and spinal cord tumors are rare, but neurologic signs are seen with cerebral xanthomas or cholesterol granulomas in geckos, green water dragons, and possibly other squamates.

Endocrine System

There are very few documented cases of endocrinopathies in reptiles. Hypothyroidism has been reported in chelonians and lizards and anecdotally linked with overfeeding of crucifers or other goitrogenic food items.

Immune System

Older animals may be more susceptible to infectious diseases, although there is little evidence to support such an assertion. In the giant tortoises, thymic hyperplasia sometimes manifests as a discrete mass at the ventral aspect of the base of the neck and may be mistaken for thyroid goiter. Thymomas are sometimes seen in older snakes, especially boa constrictors. Lymphoproliferative disorders are fairly common, especially in chelonians and snakes, and they cause clinical signs that may be very slow to progress and that vary according to the affected organ systems.

Special Senses

Lipid keratopathy, or corneal lipidosis, occurs in some agamids and iguanids and has been seen regularly in older green water dragons and plumed basilisks (*Basiliscus plumifrons*) at the Toronto Zoo. Cataracts are not uncommon in older reptiles. Age-related changes in hearing and olfactive acuity in reptiles have not been documented.

Practically all the conditions discussed are more likely to be detected early if a captive reptile is examined regularly and is followed closely by means of blood work and radiographs taken serially over the animal's life. Such assessments assist in making decisions for treatment of the individual and also allow for data to be accumulated and shared with the herpetological community, who can gradually refine their approach to diseases and care of old reptiles. Although old age cannot be cured, diagnosing age-related pathologies allows the clinician to suggest treatments and alternative husbandry methods that may improve the quality of life for aged reptiles. Older reptiles may require daily assistance to ensure adequate hydration, thermoregulation, and nutrition as they face the challenges of old age. Further, veterinary assessment combined with observations by the caregiver or owner also guides decisions about when declining quality of life may dictate euthanasia. Even if they hardly show their age, geriatric reptiles surely deserve the same attention as other geriatric animals.

REFERENCES

1. Zug GR, Vitt LJ, Caldwell JP. Tetrapod relationships and evolutionary systematics. In: Herpetology, an introductory biology of amphibians and reptiles. 2nd edition. San Diego (CA): Academic Press; 2001. p. 3–32.
2. Pough FH, Andrews RM, Cadle JE, et al. The place of amphibians and reptiles in vertebrate evolution. In: Herpetology. 2nd edition. Upper Saddle River (NJ): Prentice-Hall, Inc; 2001. p. 21–40.
3. Mader DR. Reptile medicine and surgery. Philadelphia: WB Saunders Company; 1996.

4. Girling SJ, Raiti P. BSAVA manual of reptiles. 2nd edition. Ames (IA): Blackwell Publishing; 2004.
5. Mader DR. Reptile medicine and surgery. 2nd edition. St-Louis (MO): Saunders Elsevier; 2006.
6. Kardong KV. Evolution of ageing: theoretical and practical implications from rattlesnakes. Zoo Biol 1996;15:267–77.
7. Gibbons JW. Aging phenomena in reptiles. In: Elias MF, Eleftheriou BE, Elias PK, editors. Special review of experimental aging research. Bar Harbor (ME): EAR Inc; 1976. p. 454–75.
8. Patnaik BK. Ageing in reptiles. Gerontology 1994;40:200–20.
9. Patnaik BK. Concluding remarks and future prospects. Gerontology 1994;40: 221–6.
10. Castanet J. Age estimation and longevity in reptiles. Gerontology 1994;40: 174–92.
11. Avery RA. Growth in reptiles. Gerontology 1994;40:193–9.
12. Wilson DS, Tracy CR, Tracy CR. Estimating age of turtles from growth rings: a critical evaluation of the technique. Herpetologica 2003;59:178–94.
13. Scott NM, Haussmann MF, Elsey RM, et al. Telomere length shortens with body length in *Alligator mississippiensis*. Southeast Nat 2006;5:685–92.
14. Wapstra E, Swain R, O'Reilly JM. Geographic variation in age and size at maturity in a small Australian viviparous skink. Copeia 2001;3:646–55.
15. Metcalfe NB, Monaghan P. Growth versus lifespan: perspectives from evolutionary ecology. Exp Gerontol 2003;38:935–40.
16. Carey JR, Judge DS. Longevity records: life spans of mammals, birds, amphibians, reptiles, and fish. Odense: Odense University Press; 2000.
17. Slavens F, Slavens K. Reptiles and amphibians in captivity-longevity. Available at: http://www.pondturtle.com/longev.html#INDEX. Accessed October 11, 2009.
18. Boardman W, Blanchard B. Biology, captive management, and medical care of tuatara. In: Mader DR, editor. Reptile medicine and surgery. 2nd edition. St-Louis (MO): Saunders Elsevier; 2006. p. 1008–12.
19. Lane T. Crocodilians. In: Mader DR, editor. Reptile medicine and surgery. 2nd edition. St-Louis (MO): Saunders Elsevier; 2006. p. 100–17.
20. Gibbons JW. Life in the slow lane. Nat Hist 1993;2:32.
21. Litzgus JD. Sex differences in longevity in the spotted turtle (*Clemmys guttata*). Copeia 2006;2:281–8.
22. Miller JK. Escaping senescence: demographic data from the three-toed box turtle (*Terrapene carolina triunguis*). Exp Gerontol 2001;36:829–32.
23. Metcalf AL, Metcalf EL. Longevity in some ornate box turtles (*Terrapene ornata ornata*). J Herpetol 1985;19:157–8.
24. Curtin AJ, Zug GR, Spotila JR. Longevity and growth strategies of the desert tortoise (*Gopherus agassizii*) in two American deserts. J Arid Environ 2009;73: 463–71.

Geriatric Psittacine Medicine

Teresa L. Lightfoot, DVM, DABVP-Avian

KEYWORDS

• Aging • Arthritis • Atherosclerosis • Cataracts • Neoplasia

Geriatric is defined as "related to old age." The determination that a bird is geriatric should therefore be based on knowledge of the average life expectancy of that species. Few psittacine species have been raised in captivity in significant numbers and subsequently reached geriatric status to determine at what age geriatric changes begin to occur. A preliminary table of ages for psittacine species at which they are considered geriatric has been developed, but it is anecdotal.[1] In addition, nutrition, genetics, and exercise are all major factors that can either expedite or delay changes related to aging. For purposes of discussion, geriatric is defined as the age at which medical conditions associated with aging in other species are currently being reported in psittacines.

In addition to overt disease, issues in geriatric patients include preservation of functional ability/mobility, recognizing and providing supplemental care needs, and quality of life concerns.

EVIDENCE-BASED MEDICINE

The term "evidence-based medicine" (EBM) has come into common usage in veterinary medicine, and is often used incorrectly. The consequence of this is hesitancy on the part of some veterinarians to attempt treatment when there are no controlled studies published on a given condition. If treatment is attempted, there may be concern that sharing the outcome with colleagues may lead to liability or ridicule.

The term "evidence-based medicine" is borrowed from human medicine, in which it is applied to the individual practitioner and to entire health care systems. It involves the analysis of existing data, including the critical statistical analysis of the validity of those data, as they relate to a particular treatment of a disease in a given population. As further defined by the Centre for Evidence-based Medicine, "Evidence-based medicine is the conscientious, explicit and judicious use of current best evidence in making decisions about the care of individual patients."[2] Randomized, double-blind, placebo-controlled trials involving a homogeneous patient population and medical condition are the most reliable in establishing risk versus benefit ratios and recommendations

Avian and Exotics Department, Florida Veterinary Specialists, 3000 Busch Lake Boulevard, Tampa, FL 33614, USA
E-mail address: lightfoott@aol.com

Vet Clin Exot Anim 13 (2010) 27–49
doi:10.1016/j.cvex.2009.10.002
1094-9194/10/$ – see front matter © 2010 Elsevier Inc. All rights reserved.

for patient care. However, this information is not readily available in veterinary medicine, much less in specific species of exotics.

The principles of EBM do not suggest that treatment options should not be offered in the absence of a high level of confidence in the efficacy of a drug or treatment protocol. On the contrary, the principles state that when scientific evidence is lacking, of poor quality, or conflicting, such that the risk versus benefit balance cannot be assessed, clinicians should help patients understand the uncertainty surrounding the clinical service or treatment.

Veterinarians, especially in avian medicine, seldom have the support of controlled studies in any treatment of disease conditions. A few simple guidelines should allow exploration of treatment modalities for avian patients without concern for legal ramifications or derision from colleagues. Veterinarians must be:

1. Hesitant to extrapolate from other species when a drug or treatment carries significant risk of negative side effects
2. Cognizant that in clinical practice, concurrent changes (eg, improved diet and husbandry) and tincture of time may simulate efficacy for a given treatment
3. With the owners' informed consent, willing to treat avian patients with medication and other procedures for which there is no documented species-specific efficacy or safety, when not to treat presents a greater risk, "in our best conscientious, explicit and judicious interpretation of current best evidence."

Numerous medications have been discovered inadvertently, and the method of action of many others is still unknown. A lack of research does not indicate a treatment is ineffective, only that its effectiveness is not known. Veterinarians should share their anecdotal findings (positive and negative) honestly with other veterinarians. EBM is dependent on these initial anecdotal observations for direction.[3]

WHY GERIATRIC PSITTACINES ARE ATYPICAL

The life expectancies of birds are considerably longer than those of comparably sized mammals. This fact is of research interest and relevant to veterinary care for geriatric psittacine patients.[4]

Models for Human Aging

The metabolic process in all animals produces free radicals that can damage DNA. Therefore, it is counterintuitive that birds with high metabolic rates have some of the slowest rates of senescence. Poultry and caged birds are increasingly being used as models for the study of cellular damage, including degenerative neurobiology. For instance, the enzyme telomerase allows for replacement of short pieces of DNA known as telomeres, which are otherwise lost when a cell divides. Telomerase is considered an antiaging enzyme, preventing the degradation of cell chromosomes by allowing the replacement of terminal DNA. The expression of telomerase is downregulated with age in humans. This downregulation is believed to serve as protection against neoplasia, because high telomerase activity is associated with neoplastic processes. However, in 4 species of long-lived birds tested, telomerase activity was maintained throughout the lifespan of the birds, with the longest-living birds (storm petrels) having the highest telomerase activity in most tissues tested.[5]

Although the overall incidence of neoplasia increases with age in the bird species for which there are data (poultry and quail), discrepancies between the incidences of different neoplasias in older birds may elucidate the role telomerase plays in certain types of cancer.[6]

Senility/Dementia

The effects of aging on bird cognition are unknown. Some studies have noted the effects of captivity on the hippocampus volume in birds, demonstrating that the volume is reduced in captivity, with an associated decrease in particular types of memory.[7] Cellular studies of human memory loss with aging and in human Alzheimer disease have been conducted using various avian tissues. For instance, the amyloid precursor protein (APP) is implicated in age-associated changes at synapses that contribute to memory loss in Alzheimer disease. Human and avian APP share 95% homology in amino acid sequence, and gallinaceous chicks are being used to study this protein.[8]

No controlled studies of "senility" in birds have been reported. A few anecdotal accounts from veterinarians and owners of older birds suggest that senility may occur. These reports include older birds' inability to locate entrances to cages and food sources, with which they were previously familiar, in the absence of detectable vision loss. Behavioral changes and altered interactions with long-term human and avian cohabitants are also mentioned. Changes such as these may be related to senility but also may be related to pain, discomfort, or musculoskeletal instability.

RECOGNIZING AND TREATING CHRONIC PAIN

Discussion of the frequency of various geriatric conditions should address the pain or discomfort that these conditions may cause and the disease processes themselves.

Pain studies in birds are limited. Some work has been done with nonsteroidal antiinflammatory drugs (NSAIDs), but again species variation may exist. Meloxicam (Metacam) has been shown to be readily excreted and have antiinflammatory properties in vultures and chickens, respectively.[9,10] Species variation has been demonstrated in the half-life of meloxicam, flunixin, and sodium salicylate in 5 nonpsittacine avian species.[11] Pharmacokinetics of meloxicam were performed in 1 study on psittacines, specifically ring-necked parakeets (Psittacula krameri).[12] Veterinary use of the NSAID diclofenac in South Asian cattle has resulted in a decrease in the number of 3 vulture species (Gyps spp). Vultures are exposed to diclofenac while scavenging on livestock treated with the drug shortly before death. Numerous studies have shown that diclofenac causes kidney damage, increased serum uric acid concentrations, visceral gout, and death, although meloxicam is well tolerated at comparable dosages.[13–15] Ketoprofen caused renal tubular necrosis in 1 study when used with propofol for anesthesia in eiders.[16] Flunixin meglumine (Banamine) and ketaprofen were found to be renal toxic in budgerigars.[17]

Dosages of any particular NSAID needed to achieve blood levels that are sufficient in people to block nociceptors may not be effective in any or all species of birds. The half-life of those NSAIDs tested in poultry has been only a few hours.[10] However, NSAIDs tend to migrate to sites of inflammation and are highly protein bound. Because NSAIDs block arachadonic acid from binding with the cyclooxygenase (COX) enzyme, thereby preventing conversion to thromboxane B_2, measurements of thromboxane levels may be a better assay for duration of NSAID activity. In at least 1 study, ketoprofen and flunixin administration suppressed thromboxane levels for up to 12 hours in budgerigars (Melopsittacus undulatus).[17]

Work done with synthetic opioid comparisons in psittacines has demonstrated that κ-opioid agonists such as butorphanol (Torbutrol) are superior to the μ agonists such as buprenorphine (Buprenex), although 1 study in chickens demonstrated isoflurane-sparing effects of both opioid types.[18,19] Medications such as tramadol are being used empirically in birds, but the dosage needed to affect analgesia is not known. Tramadol is a synthetic opioid that seems to have activity at the μ-opioid receptors and the noradrenergic and serotonergic systems. Therefore, the subjective efficacy of tramadol, if proven valid, may be caused by the later mechanisms. The duration of tramadol plasma levels, which in humans would affect analgesia, were considerably longer than butorphanol.[20]

The pharmacokinetics of butorphanol in raptors has shown that the half-life is much shorter than in mammals, and more frequent dosing must be used to maintain blood levels.[21] There was also variation in the rate of metabolism between raptor species, so caution should be used in extrapolation to psittacines. Additional work by Paul-Murphy[18] has demonstrated significant differences among psittacine species in dosages of butorphanol required to reach levels that provide analgesia.

Recent work with liposome-encapsulated butorphanol tartrate (LEBT) has demonstrated in Hispaniolan Amazons the potential for prolonged pain relief of up to 5 days.[22] For chronic pain in birds, this could be a valuable therapeutic option.

One study demonstrated that fentanyl (Duragesic) in cockatoos (*Cactua alba*) was not effective unless used at what the investigators considered a prohibitively (by volume and potential side effects) high dosage.[23]

Gabapentin has not been studied in birds, but its use in people and animals has shown promise. Anecdotal reports in psittacines indicate potential usefulness, especially with neuropathic pain. Studies in humans have shown variable results when gabapentin is combined with other analgesics. Most studies have demonstrated that combining gabapentin with narcotics or opioids may be useful, but combination with NSAIDs (including meloxicam) did not have a synergistic affect.[24–27]

DISEASE CONDITIONS BY SYSTEM
Special Senses: Vision, Hearing and Olfaction

Except for vision, few studies have been performed on the effects of aging on psittacine special senses. To determine the potential for aging changes to affect a particular sense significantly, the degree of development of that special sense in the bird must be determined.

Vision

Psittacines have greater visual acuity than do humans. Their range of visible light includes the ultraviolet (UV) spectrum. This UV light detection is likely involved in sexual displays, mate determination, and assessment of the ripeness of fruits. Vision loss is a life-threatening handicap in wild birds, but not necessarily in captive birds. Blind birds that have gradually lost their vision acclimate well if their caging is not altered.

Cataracts are a leading cause of blindness in older pet birds. Incipient cataracts can be easily missed without a careful ophthalmic examination. If cataract surgery is considered, an electroretinogram (ER) is advisable. Recent work with Hispaniolan Amazons has established some baselines for psittacine ER normal values.[28] Whether extracapsular extraction or phacoemulsification is preferable is controversial, and the decision should be left to the ophthalmologist performing the procedure. With either technique, the small size of the avian eye is the limiting factor. Anterior uveitis does not often occur post cataract surgery in birds, and therefore if the procedure is successful, the prognosis for restored vision is good.

Birds with monocular vision (which includes psittacines) when suffering vision loss in 1 eye tend to hold their heads so that their good eye is forward. Unilateral blindness and this prolonged positional compensation can cause scoliosis in these individuals.[29]

Iris atrophy is a common aging change in older dogs and cats and is reported in psittacines. On examination, irregular pupil margins, strands of iris that span across portions of the pupil, or holes in the stroma may be seen. Iris color change may also occur. Incomplete pupillary light reflexes are easier to detect in dogs and cats because of the absence of voluntary pupillary control, but decreased pupillary constriction may be subjectively noted in psittacines with iris atrophy. This constriction may cause light sensitivity and retinal damage.

Nuclear sclerosis (NS) occurs as an aging change in humans, dogs, cats, psittacines, and most other species of vertebrate. The nucleus of the lens becomes increasingly dense as fibers are sequentially produced and the central fibers are compressed. When the pupil is dilated, the nucleus seems gray and homogeneous. Vision affectation in animals is not generally significant. As with dogs and cats, it may be difficult without indirect ophthalmologic examination for veterinarians to differentiate NS from a cataract, and examination by an ophthalmologist is recommended. When vision loss is present but only NS is detected, retinal disease is likely.

Retinal degeneration can occur as a result of nutritional, congenital, traumatic, or viral conditions. Genetic retinal disease has been identified in commercial poultry flocks, and produced experimentally. No genetic retinal disease has yet been identified in psittacines. In people, age-related retinal (macular) degeneration occurs in 2 forms. The dry form is the most prevalent (90%) form in people. The wet form, however, accounts for most impairment of vision in humans. Birds have no true macula and age-related degeneration of the fovea has not been reported in the literature, but may occur. Darkening of the fovea in older psittacines has been reported by ophthalmologists (McNabb N and Karpinski LG, Florida, personal communication, 2009).

Pituitary tumors have been documented in birds that have presented with blindness as the primary clinical sign. These tumors are generally space-occupying adenomas (see section on Neoplastic Diseases).[30,31]

Atherosclerosis is a common condition in older pet psittacines and is discussed separately in the section on the cardiovascular system. Birds are sometimes noted to be functionally blind following an acute neurologic "episode" that causes impairment of the central nervous system, including blindness. At post mortem, these birds may have evidence of atherosclerotic plaques. In people, atherothrombotic stroke is the most common type of stroke. Size and equipment constraints currently prohibit accurate antemortem diagnosis of atherosclerosis or atherosclerotic stroke in birds.

Examination of the eyes of geriatric birds by an ophthalmologist often reveals subclinical disease. In the past 5 years, with in-house access to veterinary ophthalmologists, the following additional ocular diseases have been detected in this author's practice when a geriatric avian patient presented for a possible cataract or an annual examination: keratoconjunctivitis sicca, corneal ulceration, acquired third eyelid abnormalities, hypopyon, anterior uveitis, conjunctival granulomas, and infectious diseases involving the conjunctiva, Harderian gland adenoma, and lymphoma.

Glaucoma does occur in birds, although diagnosis in psittacines is difficult because of the size of the cornea. Most reports of normal intraocular pressures, and increased intraocular pressures indicating glaucoma, are from larger raptor species.[32]

Hearing

The hearing ability of psittacines differs from that of humans, but cannot be categorized simply as better or worse. Birds can distinguish frequencies in some ranges more accurately than can humans. These ranges are usually comparable to the range in which normal vocalizations of their species occur. However, the ability of birds to differentiate between intensities of sound or (with the exception of nocturnal predators) to localize the origin of sound is on average inferior to that of humans.

Birds may not have age-related hearing loss as is commonly seen in people. In humans, much hearing loss associated with aging is caused by loss of function of hair cells. In birds, these hair cells are able to regenerate.[33,34]

Olfaction

Historically, it was believed that birds had poor olfactory ability. Evidence involving the olfactory receptors and olfactory bulb in multiple species of birds has shown that there is a higher percentage of functional olfactory receptors in birds compared with mammals, correlating with an increased olfactory bulb capacity.[35–37] Pelagic birds and some species of vulture have specific but highly developed senses of smell. Further research is needed, but it seems that the sense of smell is more highly developed in at least some psittacine bird species, including the galah (*Eolophus roseicapillus*) and the kakapo (*Strigops habroptilus*), than was assumed previously.[36,37]

It is not known whether decreased olfactory acuity occurs in birds as they age. If it does, as with decreased visual acuity, the geriatric bird could be limited in identification of food and recognition of familiar people, birds, and objects.

Musculoskeletal

Arthritis

There are few published reports of osteoarthritic changes that have been documented radiographically in pet birds. However, limitations of range of motion in our older psittacine birds are commonly noted in practice.

In attempting to identify causes and treatments for osteoarthritis in people, mammalian models have not demonstrated the development of this condition with sufficient frequency to be useful. Studies of avian skeletons from museum collections have demonstrated that birds show an incidence of osteoarthritis similar to that of people.[38] An inverse relationship between the body weight of birds and the incidence of osteoarthritis has also been documented.[39]

Why the discrepancy between osteoarthritis documented in pet birds and the incidence that is reported in clinical practice? First, older birds are often sedentary, and abnormalities of gait are not so obvious as they are in quadruped dogs and cats. The amount of bony proliferation that accompanies arthritis in birds may also be less than that seen in mammals, particularly dogs, in which severe hip arthritis and degenerative joint disease are readily apparent on radiographs. It has been shown that osteomyelitis in birds produces less bony proliferation than is produced in mammals.[40] In addition to a less proliferative response, pet birds are smaller and therefore details of the joints are difficult to visualize with routine radiography. The hock (tibiotarsal/tarsometatarsal) joint and the stifle seem to be the most affected,[23] although coxofemoral joint range-of-motion limitations are commonly noted in older birds. Moreover, tendon calcification has been noted on histopathology of birds.[41] Tendon calcification may cause the same clinical presentation as arthritis in birds, without prominent radiographic findings.

The weight of the bird, its general physical condition, previous injuries, and any concurrent medical conditions can all contribute to the onset and severity of arthritis. Pododermatitis is often present, likely a cause and a result of decreased activity. Arthritis in 1 leg often leads to pododermatitis on the contralateral foot. Malnutrition, which decreases the integrity of the plantar epithelium, and concurrent obesity are often noted in affected birds. The cage environment, especially the variety, diameter, and texture of perches, can be important in providing comfort and stability for arthritic birds, and preventing or minimizing pododermatitis. Severely arthritic birds may need a padded platform or perch to maintain their balance. Ease of food and water access should be ensured. If the feet and nails are anatomically and positionally normal, the nails should be left with sharp points to add strength and stability to the grip. Wings should not be excessively clipped, so they can be used to help maintain balance. In addition to adjustments in the enclosure, NSAIDs such as meloxicam are being used in birds to decrease inflammation and discomfort.

Articular gout
Articular gout occurs most commonly in older psittacine birds. The onset is often acute, and increased plasma uric acid level usually accompanies the clinical presentation.

   Uric acid accumulates in the joint capsules and tendon sheaths of the joints. The metatarsophalangeal or interphalangeal joints are generally affected, and typically exhibit white to light-yellow swellings that seem grossly similar to abscesses. These uric acid deposits are painful in most birds. The cause in psittacines is generally underlying renal pathology. Treatment is discussed in the section on renal disease.

Osteoporosis
Among the causes of osteoporosis are increased phosphorus intake, calcium and vitamin D_3 deficiencies, and reduced physical activity. Deficiencies are often seen in adult female birds that are reproductively active. In older birds of either sex, osteoporosis from prolonged poor diet and inactivity is common. All seed diets provide excessive dietary phosphorus leading to insufficient calcium absorption. Radiographs may suggest osteopenia. Plasma calcium, ionized calcium, and vitamin D (specifically 25-hydroxycholecalciferol) plasma levels aid in determining appropriate therapy. Research has shown that all bird species tested to date benefit from and use oral and UV-B delivered vitamin D_3; however; African gray parrots (*Psittacus erithacus*) have a greater dependence on UV-B light for maintaining adequate serum calcium levels than do *Amazona* spp.[42]

Gastrointestinal (see Neoplastic Diseases)

Except for neoplastic disease, few conditions of the avian gastrointestinal (GI) tract have been associated with aging. Chronic vitamin A deficiency leads to squamous metaplasia along the length of the upper GI tract. Ulceration of the mucosa of the proventriculus and ventriculus can occur. These lesions may be associated with foreign bodies, known disease-causing organisms, opportunistic organisms, or no identifiable infectious or mechanical agent. Birds that have intermittent regurgitation and anorexia, and a decreased GI transit time noted on a barium series, may clinically improve when treated with H2 blockers or proton pump inhibitors. The underlying cause or causes of GI ulceration in many cases are unknown.

Cloacal disease in older birds
Intermittent cloacal bleeding in older birds is often caused by cloacal masses including papillomatosis, benign masses and polyps, and neoplastic conditions (see sections on Reproductive and Neoplastic Diseases).

Hepatic

Hepatic lipidosis is most common in obese birds on a diet that contains excess fat and is deficient in biotin, choline, and methionine. Excessive fat intake leads to lipid accumulation in hepatocytes. Mild lipidosis may be reversed. Severe and long-standing hepatic lipidosis creates a cycle of hepatocellular damage, fibrosis, and cirrhosis.

   Chronic liver disease is a common finding in older birds. Causes have not been documented for psittacines, but the history often includes obesity (and therefore potential hepatic lipidosis), probable exposure to mycotoxins, and deficiencies in vitamin A and certain amino acids. Bile acid increase is often present, with or without concurrent increases in hepatic enzymes. Serial hepatic biopsies of these birds demonstrate a progression from fibrosis to cirrhosis, with an increasing percentage of involved hepatocytes (Reavill DR, personal communication, 2008).

When the bird is no longer anorexic, dietary change is critical. Medical therapy may delay the progression of chronic liver disease to end-stage hepatic fibrosis. The efficacy of antifibrotic medication in birds is poorly documented and most is extrapolated from either human or canine/feline medicine. One mainstay of mammalian antiinflammatory therapy is corticosteroids. The risk versus benefit ratio of glucocorticoids for this use in birds has not been established.

Colchicine is used in birds as an antiinflammatory agent for articular gout and to prevent hepatic fibrosis. Numerous studies have been performed in laboratory rats that demonstrate the ability of colchicine to limit hepatic fibrosis.[43] Although there is no documentation of the efficacy of colchicine in birds, anecdotal reports suggest that it may reduce fibrosis.

Ursodeoxycholic acid (UDCA) (Ursodiol, Actigall) therapy may be beneficial in the treatment of birds with liver disease, especially those with bile acid increases. Birds produce cholic, allocholic, and chenodeoxycholic acids, which can produce hepatocellular lysis. UDCA may replace these bile acids and promote bile excretion. This drug is the first-line treatment for humans with biliary cirrhosis. Its immune-modulating effects may also be beneficial in hepatic inflammatory conditions. Again, dosages are extrapolated from human or small mammal medicine and efficacy is unproven.

HEPATIC NEOPLASIA (SEE NEOPLASTIC DISEASES)
Renal

Renal disease is present in a high percentage of birds at necropsy, and has few noninvasive definitive tests available ante mortem. Uric acid increase can indicate renal disease, but can also be a function of diet or contamination. Normal uric acid levels do not exclude renal functional impairment.

Obtaining and interpreting a urinalysis is difficult because of fecal comingling in the cloaca and the lack of a urinary bladder. The presence of proteinuria in birds may be a result of fecal contamination. Conversely, the absence of proteinuria may be caused by the absence of proteolytic enzymes in avian leukocytes, so that protein-losing nephropathy may not occur in avian glomerular disease.[44]

Older birds on a lifelong deficient diet may have an adverse reaction when suddenly placed on a balanced pelleted diet. This reaction may be noted as polyuria/polydipsia (PU/PD) or general malaise, with possible increase of plasma uric acid levels. One theory for this occurrence is that the renal (and often hepatic) parenchyma is reduced in function because of chronic deficiencies in vitamin A precursors and amino acids (lysine, methionine, and cysteine, among others). This parenchyma seems to be most common in cockatiels. These birds may already have compromised renal function caused by chronic malnutrition (ie, squamous metaplasia of the tubules and collecting ducts of the kidney from chronic vitamin A deficiency may cause renal tubular disease). The desquamated metaplastic squamous epithelial cells can obstruct urinary production and flow. Change to a pelleted diet that contains higher, albeit "normal" levels of protein, may overload their compromised renal and hepatic capacities. Therefore, caution should be used in improving the diet of geriatric birds, even when plasma chemistries are normal. Often, the gradual addition of a quality pelleted diet with close observation of the bird's fecal and urinary output, attitude, and weight, allow the owner and veterinarian to determine whether a complete or partial conversion to a pelleted diet can be achieved in a geriatric avian patient.

Renal biopsy is the best method of determining the presence, type, and extent of renal disease. Histopathologic diagnoses of nephrosis (urate or other), bacterial nephritis, glomerulopathy, or fibrosis, all change the treatment of the bird and its prognosis. A renal biopsy obtained endoscopically on a stable avian patient by a practitioner experienced in this technique carries a minimal risk.[44] If renal biopsy is not possible, older birds presenting for PU/PD, nonspecific clinical signs of lethargy, with normal blood glucose levels, increased or "high normal" fasting uric acid levels, mild anemia, and a persistent heterophilia may warrant treatment of renal disease.

Treatment of the various conditions of the kidney that may be determined via biopsy have been published elsewhere.[44] Pending biopsy results, antibiotics are warranted for potential bacterial nephritis. In most cases, omega-3 fatty acids are valuable and have been shown to decrease inflammation and increase renal vascular flow and glomerular filtration rates.[45] The use of antiinflammatory agents such as aspirin, colchicine, allopurinol, and probenecid may be considered. The use of aggressive fluid therapy initially and long-term diuresis may be an important part of treatment in psittacine renal disease, depending on the cause of the disease and the response of the bird to the fluid therapy.

The feasibility of continued fluids at home must take into account the owner's willingness and the temperament of the bird. In 1 ongoing case, this author's practice has monitored a Goffin cockatoo (*Cacatua goffini*) with renal nephrosis, after initial hospitalization and diagnostics, for more than 18 months while it has received at-home administration of subcutaneous fluids (and omega-3 fatty acids and a low protein pelleted diet). In this individual (and not uncommonly in this genus of psittacine) the bird is complacent for the treatment and forgiving following treatment. For most species of the genera *Amazona* and *Ara*, unless the owner is unusually adept at administration, the outlook for fluid therapy administered by the owner yet maintaining the owner-pet bond is less positive (see section on Administration of Medications).

Treatment of articular gout may be unrewarding. Colchicine and allopurinol are used as antiinflammatory agents. Aggressive fluid therapy may be attempted, and dietary supplementation with omega-3 fatty acids and vitamin A precursors. Probenecid usage is controversial in avian gout.[46] Pain relief may be attempted by frequent administration of butorphanol. It is to be hoped that, with further research, the long-acting liposome-encapsulated butorphanol will continue to demonstrate a long half-life in the avian system of various species and become commercially available. Caution should be used in prescribing NSAIDs in these birds because of the potential for renal compromise. Because of the pain displayed by birds with uncontrolled articular gout, if pain cannot be controlled, euthanasia should be considered.

Endocrine

Reports of endocrine diseases in older birds other than neoplasia are not common. An adrenal syndrome of vacuolation of the interrenal cells (the equivalent of the mammalian adrenal cortical cells) is seen in African gray parrots (*Psittacus erithacus*), often resulting in sudden death.[30]

Pancreatic islet cell hyperplasia has been noted occasionally on histopathology. The A cells (which secrete glucagon) are most often affected. If there is a correlation with hyperglycemia in psittacines, it has not been documented; clinical signs reported with necropsy submissions for histopathology have been vague.

Hyperglycemia (avian diabetes mellitus) is not uncommon in mature, obese birds and in females that have had prolonged hyperestrogenism. Moderately increased glucose levels (700–800 mg/dL or 40 mmol/L) may be transient hyperglycemia and not representative of a primary diabetes mellitus.

Hypertrophy of the parathyroid glands is noted in birds that chronically consume a diet insufficient in calcium. These birds may also demonstrate bony lesions at necropsy.[41]

Nonneoplastic diseases of the thyroid gland in psittacines are poorly understood. Autoimmune thyroiditis has been documented in poultry but not in psittacines. Degenerative thyroid lesions are reported occasionally on histopathology, but the cause is unknown. The incidence of hypothyroidism in psittacines is also unknown, likely because of the historical lack of availability of thyroid-stimulating hormone for testing.

Cardiovascular

As birds live longer and diagnostics improve, a greater incidence of avian cardiac disease is being detected. Cardiac disease can still be difficult to diagnose and may mimic other conditions, such as respiratory, hepatic, or ovarian disease. The bird may present in a weak or lethargic condition or with increased respiratory rate and effort. With right-sided heart disease, hepatomegaly and ascites are common. Disease may also be subclinical, then present acutely, and the bird may expire when diagnostics or treatment are attempted. Right heart disease is more prevalent in birds than left-sided cardiac disease, as discussed later.

Pulmonary hypertension

The avian cardiovascular system differs anatomically and physiologically from the mammalian in several parameters. The physiologic responses that maintain low pulmonary vascular resistance in mammals (vascular distensibility and vasculature recruitment) are absent in birds,[47] which results in the inability of the pulmonary vasculature to accommodate increased cardiac output by either altering vessel diameter or changing the percentage of vasculature channels being used. This result is, at least in part, responsible for the high incidence of pulmonary hypertension syndrome (PHS) in the poultry industry and right-sided heart disease in psittacine patients.

Because of the financial impact of PHS in broiler hens, much research has been conducted in this area. In addition to the lack of vascular accommodation in avian species as noted earlier, studies have demonstrated that the response to pulmonary arterial hypertension in chickens is an increase in 2 vasoactive substances, the vasodilator nitric oxide (NO) and the vasoconstrictor serotonin 5-hydroxytryptamine (5-HT); the vasoconstrictor 5-HT predominates over the vasodilator NO in broiler hens susceptible to PHS.[48] For the broiler industry, genetic selection of hens is being investigated. For geriatric psittacine patients, this would indicate that specific vasodilator therapy in cases of pulmonary hypertension might be of value and warrants further research. The avian anatomy makes visualizing the pulmonary artery and vein via echocardiology difficult.[49] Also, even if indirect measurements of avian systemic blood pressure (BP) become reliable to obtain, they do not directly correlate with pulmonary pressures.

Although it is a subjective parameter, birds whose jugular veins become extremely distended when gently occluded for venipuncture are often the same patients (commonly African gray parrots [Psittacus erithacus]) that have the signalment for pulmonary hypertension and atherosclerosis. The use of angiotensin-converting enzyme (ACE) inhibitors such as enalapril (Enacard) and benazepril (Lotensin) and inodilators such as pimobendan (Vetmedin) may be considered in these patients, with the caveats of unproven efficacy and unknown risk.

Macaw asthma
Macaw asthma, or macaw polycythemia, may theoretically cause pulmonary hypertension, from chronic air capillary hypoxia and subsequent polycythemia. No published data on pulmonary hypertension in macaws diagnosed with this syndrome were located.

Renal shunt and cardiovascular disease
Another potential cause of cardiac disease in birds is the existence of the renal portal shunt, which allows bacteria from the lower GI tract to enter the general circulation without filtration by the liver.[50] This increased chance of bacterial sepsis may lead to a higher incidence of valvular and thromboembolic disease.

Epicardial and myocardial fat
In chronically obese birds, epicardial fat and infiltration of fat into the myocardium is seen at necropsy. The clinical history of these birds often includes sudden death, with no other significant findings on gross or histopathologic examination.[51]

Atherosclerosis
Atherosclerosis is common in psittacine birds. It is generally a geriatric condition,[52] with the exception of African gray parrots (*Psittacus erithacus*), in which this disease has been noted with some frequency in younger animals. The most common sign is sudden death; in people, coronary, carotid artery, and peripheral vascular occlusions from atherosclerosis are often not diagnosed until the conditions are well advanced. Without the ability to perform cardiac catheterization and concurrent measurement of vessel diameters, antemortem diagnosis in psittacines is unlikely.[53] Other diagnostic modalities including duplex ultrasound, magnetic resonance imaging, and angiography are generally cost and size prohibitive in psittacine birds.

Clinical signs may include dyspnea, lethargy, paresis, blindness, ataxia, or collapse. Tentative diagnosis is based on:

1. Increased risk factors such as age, species, obesity, dietary history, and inactivity
2. Blood work findings that include lipemic serum, increased plasma cholesterol levels, increased triglycerides, increased low-density lipoproteins (LDLs) and decreased high-density lipoproteins (HDLs)
3. Chronic egg-laying birds with estrogen-induced lipemia (note: in the avian liver, estrogen causes the conversion of carbohydrate to triglyceride and the production of proteins involved in the production of triglyceride-rich lipoprotein particles, leading to hypersecretion of these lipoproteins into the circulation[54])
4. Clinical signs such as episodic dyspnea, lethargy, paresis, blindness, ataxia, or collapse
5. Radiographic evidence of calcification and widening of the greater vessels, most commonly the right aortic arch, or cardiomegaly.

These clinical and laboratory findings are anecdotal or extrapolated from human medicine. Definitive research in causation, diagnosis, and treatment of atherosclerosis in psittacines is lacking. In birds, atherosclerosis most commonly affects the aorta and brachiocephalic trunks. The coronary arteries are less often affected; therefore ischemia of the myocardium is uncommon. Numerous cases of atherosclerosis in psittacines have been published.[55–60]

As in people, weight loss, increased activity, and dietary regulation are all in line with improvement of overall health and presumed preventative measures against atherosclerotic plaques. In some cases, practitioners may elect to institute therapy with lipid-lowering medications such as statins. No dosages are available for birds, nor are any given in this article, but extrapolation from human medicine (accounting for the higher metabolism of birds) is being used for dosing. Anecdotal reports, including patients from this author's practice, have had significant reductions in cholesterol and triglycerides that did not occur with diet change alone. No adverse affects have been noted in the limited cases available. Nor can it be stated definitively that these drugs have been effective in preventing atherosclerosis. One study has shown that ginseng is effective in lowering plasma cholesterol levels in birds.[61]

Echocardiology

The response to the stress of handling can increase heart rate and oxygen demand significantly in birds; therefore, inhalant anesthesia is preferred to manual restraint for performance of echocardiograms in all but the most docile patients. Equipment recommendations include an ultrasound unit with Doppler function, 100 frames/s minimum speed and microcurved or phased array probes with minimum 7.5 MHz frequency. Anatomic constraints in birds also limit the echocardiographic windows available. Parameters for chamber sizes, blood flow velocities, functional contractility, and valvular insufficiency have been determined for several species and studies are ongoing.[42] In birds with decreased myocardial contractility and reduced fractional shortening, anecdotal reports of a positive response to enalapril are common. When right-sided cardiac insufficiency and ascites are present, furosemide has been clinically useful in treatment.

The avian veterinarian is advised to work in conjunction with a cardiologist on avian patients with suspected cardiac disease. Diagnosis of the cardiovascular abnormality and formulation of a therapeutic plan require knowledge of avian anatomy and physiology and the cardiologist's diagnostic skills and pharmacologic recommendations. Although most avian therapeutic regimes are still extrapolated from mammalian regimes, numerous reports indicate that cardiac drug therapy can improve cardiac function, thereby increasing the quality and length of the life of the bird. Furosemide, enalapril, and pimobendin have all been used to treat avian cardiac disease. No controlled studies of the effects of these drugs are available.

Indirect BP measurements

In 1 study of 16 healthy Amazon parrots, no correlation was found between direct and indirect BP readings.[62] Other practitioners have reported anecdotal correlation between BP and clinical signs of hypertension. BP measurements in psittacines would be valuable in treatment of septic shock, blood loss, cardiac disease, renal disease, and atherosclerosis, along with monitoring avian patients during anesthesia. However, until further studies are conducted that determine an accurate indirect method of measuring BP in psittacines, BP measurements should be at best considered as trends in the individual patient.[62]

Arrhythmias

Second-degree atrioventricular (AV) block has been reported anecdotally and in a recent case report.[63] However, there has not been documentation in psittacines that cardiac arrhythmias are noted more commonly in older birds, nor of a physiologic trigger or pathologic cause. Whether arrhythmias are truly less common in psittacines than in mammals or more difficult to detect via auscultation and electrocardiogram (ECG) because of the rapid heart rate, is not known.

Reproductive

Decreased reproductive success has been noted with aging in all species tested. Although poultry studies predominate, in aging hens a decreased clutch number, decreased frequency of clutches, and decreased viability of young have been documented in other birds such as swans and multiple zoologic species.[53]

Cystic ovaries

The frequency of cystic ovarian disease in mature and aging psittacine hens is unknown. It has been reported anecdotally and by avian pathologists.[64] Tentative diagnosis is often via radiology or ultrasound. This condition may occur alone or in conjunction with other reproductive pathology, such as egg yolk peritonitis and ovarian neoplasia. Cystic ovarian disease may be asymptomatic, or present in various ways. Breeding behavior in the absence of egg laying, increased sternopubic distance, abdominal distention, and subsequent dyspnea from coelomic mass effect are possible clinical signs. Ovocentesis for relief of the space-occupying effect and for differentiation between cystic ovarian disease and infection may be accomplished with ultrasound guided aspiration. Leuprolide acetate (Depo-Lupron) has been used to stimulate follicular atresia. In many cases of documented cystic ovaries, the presence or absence of concurrent ovarian disease or neoplasia has not been determined.

Gonadotropin inhibitory hormone (GnIH) synthesis and GnIH receptors have been isolated in the avian reproductive system, including ovarian granulosa cells, along with the interstitial layer and seminiferous tubules of the testis in studies on 2 orders of birds: Passeriformes and Galliformes.[65] This mechanism may provide an alternate treatment of ovarian cysts and induce cessation of breeding behavior if the hormone becomes commercially available.

Egg yolk peritonitis, egg yolk stroke, and oviductal prolapse are reproductive diseases that may persist in older birds, but are primarily diseases of mature adult hens.

Neoplastic Diseases

Statistics on the rate of occurrence of various neoplasias in birds are usually obtained from the files of avian and exotic veterinary pathologists. Few practitioners or institutions have sufficient caseloads to develop meaningful statistics. The data published by pathologists are useful and would be made more so if practitioners who submit samples provided more extensive histories.

Xanthomas

Xanthomas are generally friable, yellow-colored fatty-appearing masses that may be located anywhere on the body, but are often seen on the distal wing, in the sternopubic area, and on the keel. The origin of xanthomas is unknown; however, dietary improvement, including sufficient vitamin A or vitamin A precursors, has been noted to be curative in less advanced cases.[66] Xanthomas tend to be vascular and surgical excision, when necessary, should be undertaken with due attention to hemostasis. Diffuse xanthomas may be amenable to cryotherapy, but attention must be paid to maintenance of the vascular supply.[67]

Lipomas

Lipomas occur most frequently in budgerigars, but are also seen in *Amazona* spp, *Ara* spp, cockatiels (*Nymphicus hollandicus*), and other psittacines, and are often associated with excessive body fat. These masses are usually located on the keel or in the sternopubic area. Malignant liposarcomas are rare in psittacines.[68]

In older psittacines, xanthomas and lipomas may become life threatening when they are present in the sternopubic area. Concurrent abdominal herniation is often present, and when combined with an extensive mass, may result in difficulty in evacuation of the cloaca, abrasion, hemorrhage, and infection. A combination of weight loss, altered environment to prevent trauma to the area, and surgery may be required. The practitioner must bear in mind that these older birds often have hepatic lipidosis, decreased hepatic function, coagulopathies, and cardiovascular disease. Surgery, if necessary, should be as kept as noninvasive and as short duration as is possible.

If the bird is a good candidate for abdominal surgery, a GI contrast study or ultrasound should be performed to determine if bowel loops are present in the herniated sternopubic area before surgical intervention.

Fibrosarcomas

Fibrosarcomas can occur anywhere on the body, but are most commonly seen on the face, in the oral cavity, associated with long bones, or in the abdominal cavity. They tend to be locally invasive and often recur with conservative surgical excision. Local treatment with radiation therapy is often indicated for providing long-term control. The metastatic rate is low, so local disease management is paramount.[67] Surgical excision followed by radiation and chemotherapy has been reported with some success. Strontium radiation therapy, although limited by depth of penetration, has been anecdotally reported as efficacious in several instances.

Squamous cell carcinomas

Squamous cell carcinomas (SCC) may also occur anywhere on the body, being most prevalent at mucocutaneous junctions, in the oral cavity, in the infraorbital sinus, on the distal wing, the phalanges, and the uropygial gland.[69] SCC tend to be aggressively locally invasive, and complete excision is rarely accomplished. Radiation therapy has been attempted with some success; however, SCC seems to be an exceptionally radioresistant tumor and long-term control is rare. Anecdotal reports indicate that radioresistance may be greater in birds than in mammals. Strontium therapy when tumor depth is not a limiting factor has shown some promise in selected psittacine cases. Distant metastasis is rare; therefore systemic chemotherapy is not commonly used. Photodynamic therapy has been attempted in 2 reported cases. One case of SCC in the beak of a hornbill showed a positive result in decreasing tumor size but failure to eliminate the neoplasia.[70] Other case reports had equivocal results.[71] Intralesional cisplatin and intralesional cisplatin combined with cryosurgery have been effective in inducing partial remissions in 3 cases of oral and 1 case of submandibular SCC in psittacines in this author's practice. Species involved included a 26-year-old Congo African gray (Psittacus erithacus), an 8-year-old male Eclectus sp, a green wing macaw more than 30 years old (Ara chloroptera) and a 36-year-old Wagler's conure (Aratinga wagleri) (Maldonado, Lightfoot, Stevenson, unpublished data). Although to the author's knowledge, age-related data have not been collated, SCC seems to occur with greater frequency in geriatric psittacines. The constant necrosis caused by the SCC itself and by the chemo- and cryotherapies produce a fertile breeding ground for bacteria, yeast, and fungus. Appropriate antimicrobial therapy should be continued throughout the duration of treatment to avoid septicemia.

Melanomas

Melanomas are not common in birds, but are 1 of the few tumors in which distant metastasis is noted. Primary malignant melanoma has been diagnosed on the beak, in the liver, on the skin of the face, and in the oral cavity of psittacines. Metastatic melanoma lesions have been noted in the cardiac muscle, kidneys, and brain. Aggressive local invasion of a malignant melanoma was also seen in the sinus of an African gray parrot (Psittacus erithacus).[71] Ages of birds involved have not been reported.

Musculoskeletal system

Chondroma, hemangioma, and malignant tumors including osteosarcoma, chondrosarcoma, and leiomyosarcoma have all been reported. Wide surgical resection or amputation are the suggested methods of treatment, as benign lesions are often cured with complete excision and a decrease in tumor burden can be accomplished in malignant lesions. Extrapolation from canine and feline oncology may suggest other modalities, such as radiation therapy for additional local treatment and chemotherapy for systemic control.[67]

A biopsy should be obtained from patients in which radiographic bony lesions are present. Under inhalant anesthesia, a 23- to 20-gauge needle can be surgically introduced into the bone. A sufficient sample is usually obtained and subsequently retained in the hub of the needle. The sample can them be dislodged with smaller gauge wire and submitted.

Internal carcinomas

Ovarian neoplasias (various cell origins), renal carcinomas, hepatic adenocarcinoma, hepatobiliary and pancreatic adenocarcinoma, splenic, and gastric carcinomas have all been reported in older psittacines.

A few case reports and anecdotal reports exist indicating intralesional cisplatin or carboplatin therapy may be useful in ovarian and renal adenocarcinoma, generally following surgical debulking and confirmation of the neoplasia via histopathology.[72,73] Bile duct carcinoma has also been treated with carboplatin successfully in 1 report.[74] Toxicity studies with cisplatin and carboplatin in cockatoos indicate that psittacine tolerance for these drugs may be greater than that of mammals.[75,76]

Ovarian neoplasia

Similar to human ovarian adenocarcinoma, p53 tumor suppressor gene alterations are common in chicken ovarian adenocarcinomas and correlate with the number of lifetime ovulations.[77] Aspirin treatment may inhibit the progression of ovarian cancer in the hen.[78]

Tamoxifen has been used for its antiestrogen effect in chicken ovaries in dozens of studies relating to human female reproduction. One study conducted in budgerigars demonstrated minimal side effects of tamoxifen administration, the main one being leucopenia. Although the study was designed to assess safety, the change in cere color of the hens from brown to blue implies that estrogen was inhibited.[79–81] GnRH agonists have been effective empirically; however, confirmation of neoplasia (as opposed to cystic ovarian disease) has often not been obtained.

Gastric, biliary, hepatic, and pancreatic neoplasias

Gastric carcinomas can be seen in the esophagus and most commonly at the proventricular/ventricular junction. There is an apparent predilection for this neoplasia in *Amazonas* spp, and budgerigars (*Melopsittacus undulates*).[82] Diagnosis can be difficult, because they tend to be flat to ulcerative lesions (not proliferative). Radiographic GI contrast studies may demonstrate an irregular mucosa and suggest a neoplastic process. Isthmus carcinomas can ulcerate through the serosa, causing coelomitis.

Biliary and pancreatic carcinomas are frequently diagnosed in the genus *Amazona* and to a lesser degree *Ara* in conjunction with internal papillomatosis.[83] The herpes virus of Pacheco disease has been identified in birds with internal papillomatosis. The genotype of the herpes virus and the species of bird contribute to susceptibility to acute Pacheco disease or the development of internal papillomatosis.[84]

Reports of various tumors in the liver of birds include hepatocellular carcinoma, cholangiocarcinoma, lipoma, sarcoma, hemangioma/sarcoma, and adenocarcinoma.

Carboplatin has been used in several cases with equivocal results, but with no apparent toxicity. Tumors that metastasize to the liver are uncommon, but include lymphoma and pancreatic carcinoma. The reported incidence of primary hepatocellular carcinoma is low in Old World species.

Endocrine neoplasias

Pituitary adenomas have been documented in multiple avian species but are most prevalent in budgerigars and cockatiels.[67] Affected animals may present with acute neurologic conditions (seizures/opisthotonos/blindness). They may also present with conditions related to the pituitary hormones that are affected. Usually, this is pronounced polydipsia and polyuria. Occasional presentations are of a retrobulbar mass and subsequent exophthalmia. In human medicine, surgical resection and radiation therapy (if needed) are used for treatment. Size and monetary constraints make routine treatment by these methods unlikely in small psittacine patients.

Lymphoma/Lymphosarcoma

Lymphoma may have many presentations in older pet birds, including lymphatic, hemopoietic, hepatic, and cutaneous lymphoma. The incidence of oral lymphosarcoma in *Amazona* spp and retrobulbar or periorbital presentations in Congo African grays (*Psittacus erithacus*) is overrepresented.[85] Chemotherapy is the treatment of choice for systemic disease. Surgery and radiation therapies have been successfully employed in cases of solitary lymphoma. To date, no evidence of retroviral activity has been associated with psittacine lymphoma.[67,85]

Respiratory Neoplasia

Primary respiratory neoplasia is uncommon in psittacines. An exception seems to be an intrathoracic neoplasia reported in cockatiels (*Nymphicus hollandicus*). It is characterized by the inclusion of 2 cell types, having mesenchymal and epithelial cell components.[86] Few other primary pulmonary neoplasias have been reported in the literature. Metastatic pulmonary neoplasia may occur, but it is not noted with the same frequency as is documented in dogs.[67,87,88]

Note Regarding Treatment of Psittacine Neoplasia

The presentation of anecdotal treatments in the literature is problematic. Preliminary information regarding clinical response may expand the practitioner's ability to attempt treatment. However, future studies may either reinforce these protocols, or demonstrate a lack of efficacy or serious side effects.

For localized tumors, when surgical excision is incomplete or impossible, alternative forms of therapy, including external beam radiation (cobalt 60 or linear accelerator), cryotherapy, photodynamic therapy, or hand-held radiation applicators bear consideration.

Rapid advances in treatment recommendations warrant a current literature search before making recommendations for therapy. Consultation with other avian veterinarians and veterinary oncologists is advisable.

ADMINISTRATION OF MEDICATION AND QUALITY OF LIFE

Many geriatric conditions discussed in this article require long-term medication. In many if not most birds, direct oral administration is a stressful event for the bird and the owner. Helping the owner to find alternatives (the most common being admixing the medication in a favorite soft food) can greatly enhance compliance and quality of life. Ideally, owners should find a favorite soft food that is given occasionally as a treat before the need for medication. The importance of this quality of life issue is often overlooked in practice.

THE GERIATRIC ANNUAL EXAMINATION

As the pet psittacine population ages, practitioners are developing long-standing relationships with the individual bird and its owner. An annual office visit and physical examination offer an opportunity to prevent overt disease processes by correcting husbandry issues and detecting early warning signs of disease. Record keeping that includes the condition of the plumage, of the plantar epithelium of the feet, grip strength, and response of the cardiovascular and respiratory systems to restraint can be as useful as laboratory tests. Minimally, these visits should include:

a. A candid discussion with the owner regarding quality of life, encompassing changes in behavior that could be manifestations of pain, nervousness, fear, or disorientation such as the extent of vocalization, play, and movement within the bird's environment, and interaction with objects, other birds and people, compared with previous years
b. Questions designed to detect incipient disease, such as changes in water consumption or urinary output, changes in food preferences or eating habits, reproductive and sexual behaviors, alterations in preening habits, changes of preferred perching locations, sleep cycle alterations
c. A thorough physical examination that includes the routine physical examination and assessment of weight, muscle mass, grip strength, joint range of motion, ambulation, flight if applicable, feather condition, and exercise tolerance
d. Radiographs to evaluate bone density, arthritic changes, cardiovascular abnormalities, organomegaly and to screen for coelomic masses
e. Complete blood count and plasma chemistries, including bile acids, triglycerides, cholesterol, and HDL and LDL levels if indicated
f. Ophthalmic examination
g. Echocardiogram and ECG if warranted.

MEDICATIONS MENTIONED IN THE TEXT

Pharmocodynamic and kinetic studies have not been completed on most medications in the following list. Those drugs preceded by a single asterisk contain studies mentioned within the body of the article. However, none have the strength of evidence to qualify for the levels of grade A (randomized controlled trials and meta-analyses) or B (other evidence such as well-designed controlled and uncontrolled studies) for multiple psittacine species.

Judicious extrapolation needs to be made from diagnostics and treatments found effective in other species. Anecdotal experiences and information should be shared with owners and colleagues to best serve current patients and to give direction to future research.

Despite the tens of thousands of psittacines imported into the United States from the 1960s to the 1980s, there is little information on geriatric parrots. Most of these parrots are dead. It is to be hoped that improvements in nutrition and husbandry will change this situation and avian veterinarians will have increasing numbers of geriatric patients. Thoughtful alterations to the aging bird's environment can increase the quality of life of geriatric psittacines when mobility is compromised or vision impaired.

Drug	Dosage	Indications	Comments
*Meloxicam	0.5–1.0 mg/kg IV, PO every 12–24 h	Pain, inflammation, SCC	Occasional GI upset
*Butorphanol tartrate	1–3 mg/kg IV, PO every 2–6 h	Pain, sedation, reduction of inhalant anesthetic level. Higher range for Amazons	Short half-life (1–2 h) in species tested. PO may not reach adequate blood levels.
*LEBT	NA to date	Patent pending, may be effective for up to 5 days	May last up to 5 days
*Buprenorphine	0.05–1.0 mg/kg every 6 – 12 h	Pain sedation, reduction of inhalant anesthetic	In chickens; efficacy still questionable in other species
*Tramadol	5 mg/kg IV or PO every 6–24 h	Pain, sedation	Limited research in birds
*Fentanyl	0.02–0.2 mg/kg SC (see Comments)**	Analgesia; not currently recommended	**Low doses ineffective; higher doses have potential complications
Colchicine	0.01–2.0 mg/kg PO every 12–24 h	Hyperuricemia, hepatic or renal inflammation or fibrosis	Note wide empirical dosage range and potential to increase uric acid levels noted in some raptors
Allopurinol	10 mg/kg PO every 24 h	Hyperuricemia	Narrow range between efficacy and toxicity in hawks
Ursodeoxycholic acid	10–15 mg/kg PO every 24 h	Biliary stasis, increased bile acids	Subjective efficacy in reducing bile acid levels
Leuprolide acetate (Depo-Lupron)	200–800 µg/kg IM every 4 weeks prn	Cystic ovarian disease, excessive egg laying, estrogen dependent ovarian neoplasia?	No controlled studies; extensive empirical reports of efficacy but dosage range subjective
Enalapril	0.25–1.0 mg/kg every 24–48 h	Cardiomyopathy	ACE inhibitor
Furosemide	0.5–2.0 mg/kg every 6–24 h	Diuretic	Species sensitivities, including lories
Pimobendin	0.1–1.0 mg/kg every 12–24 h	Pulmonary arterial dilator, cardiomyopathy	Atherosclerosis, only anecdotal reports
Atropine	0.01–0.05 mg/kg every 6–12 h	Bronchodilator, anticholinesterase	
Atropine	0.2–0.5 mg/kg	Bradycardia, cardiopulmonary resuscitation	

Abbreviations: IM, intramuscularly; IV, intravenously; NA, not applicable; PO, by mouth; prn, as required; SC, subcutaneously.

ACKNOWLEDGMENTS

The author would like to thank all her colleagues in avian medicine. The spirit of cooperation and collaboration in our niche of veterinarian medicine is a lifelong source of pride, gratification, and wonder.

REFERENCES

1. Wilson L, Lightfoot TL. Concepts in behavior: section III pubescent and adult psittacine behavior. In: Harrison GJ, Lightfoot TL, editors. Clinical avian medicine. Lake Worth (FL): Spix; 2006. p. 73–83.
2. Haussler B. [Definition, procedures and goals of evidence-based medicine]. Dtsch Med Wochenschr 2005;130(Suppl 2):S66–71.
3. Ian A. How should physicians treat evidence-based medicine? In: Ian A, editor. Super crunchers. New York: Bantam Dell; 2007. p. 88–111.
4. Mueller A. Relative longevity and field metabolic rate in birds. J Evol Biol 2008; 21(5):1379–86.
5. Haussmann MF, Winkler DW, Huntington CE, et al. Telomerase activity is maintained throughout the lifespan of long-lived birds. Exp Gerontol 2007;42(7): 610–8.
6. Swanberg SE, Delany ME. Dynamics of telomere erosion in transformed and non-transformed avian cells in vitro. Cytogenet Genome Res 2003;102(1–4):318–25.
7. Ladage LD, Fox RA, Pravosudov VV. Effects of captivity and memory-based experiences on the hippocampus in mountain chickadees. Behav Neurosci 2009;123(2):284–91.
8. Mileusnic R, Lancashire CL, Rose SP. Amyloid precursor protein: from synaptic plasticity to Alzheimer's disease. Ann N Y Acad Sci 2005;1048:149–65.
9. Naidoo V, Wolter K, Cromarty AD, et al. The pharmacokinetics of meloxicam in vultures. J Vet Pharmacol Ther 2008;31(2):128–34.
10. Baert K, De Backer P. Disposition of sodium salicylate, flunixin and meloxicam after intravenous administration in broiler chickens. J Vet Pharmacol Ther 2002; 25(6):449–53.
11. Baert K. Comparative pharmacokinetics of three non-steroidal anti-inflammatory drugs in five bird species. Comp Biochem Physiol C Toxicol Pharmacol 2003; 34(1):25–33.
12. Wilson H. Pharmacokinetics and use of Meloxicam in psittacine birds. In: AAV conference proceedings; 2004.
13. Hussain I, Khan MZ, Khan A, et al. Toxicological effects of diclofenac in four avian species. Avian Pathol 2008;37(3):315–21.
14. Naidoo V, Swan GE. Veterinary diclofenac threatens Africa's endangered vulture species. Regul Toxicol Pharmacol 2009. [Epub ahead of print].
15. Naidoo V, Swan VE. Diclofenac toxicity in Gyps vulture is associated with decreased uric acid excretion and not renal portal vasoconstriction. Comp Biochem Physiol C Toxicol Pharmacol 2009;149(3):269–74.
16. Mulcahy DM, Tuomi P, Larsen RS, et al. Differential mortality of male spectacled eiders (*Somateria fischeri*) and king eiders (*Somateria spectabilis*) subsequent to anesthesia with propofol, bupivacaine, and ketoprofen. J Avian Med Surg 2003; 17(3):117–23.
17. Pereira ME, Werther K. Evaluation of the renal effects of flunixin meglumine, ketoprofen and meloxicam in budgerigars (*Melopsittacus undulatus*). Vet Rec 2007;160(24):844–6.

18. Paul-Murphy JR. Analgesic effects of butorphanol and bupreorphine in conscious African Grey parrots (*Psittacus erithacus erithacus*). Am J Vet Res 1999;60: 1218–21.

19. Concannon KT, Hellyer PW. Influence of a mu- and kappa opioid agonist on isoflurane minimal anesthetic concentration in chickens. Vet Res 1995;56:806–11.

20. Souza MJ, Cox SA. Pharmacokinetics of tramadol in bald eagles (*Haliaeetus leucocephalus*). In: AAV conference proceedings; 2007.

21. Riggs SM, Hawkins MG, Craigmill AL, et al. Pharmacokinetics of butorphanol tartrate in red-tailed hawks (*Buteo jamaicensis*) and great horned owls (*Bubo virginianus*). Am J Vet Res 2008;69(5):596–603.

22. Sladky KK. Serum concentrations and analgesic effects of liposome-encapsulated and standard butorphanol tartrate in parrots. Am J Vet Res 2006;67(5):775–81.

23. Hoppes S. Disposition and analgesic effects of fentanyl in white cockatoos (*Cacatua alba*). J Avian Med Surg 2003;17(3):124–30.

24. Gilron I, Orr E, Dongsheng T, et al. A randomized, double-blind, controlled trial of perioperative administration of gabapentin, meloxicam and their combination for spontaneous and movement-evoked pain after ambulatory laparoscopic cholecystectomy. Anesth Analg 2009;108(2):623–30.

25. Devor M. How does gabapentin relieve neuropathic pain? Pain 2009;45(1–2): 259–61.

26. de Medicis E. Gabapentin and post-thoracotomy shoulder pain. Can J Anaesth 2008;55(12):878–9, author reply 879.

27. Davis JL, Posner LP, Elce Y. Gabapentin for the treatment of neuropathic pain in a pregnant horse. J Am Vet Med Assoc 2007;231(5):755–8.

28. Hendrix DVH, Sims MH. Electroretinography in the Hispaniolan Amazon Parrot (*Amazona ventralis*). J Avian Med Surg 2004;18(2):89–94.

29. Turhan E, Acaroglu E, Bozkurt G, et al. Unilateral enucleation affects the laterality but not the incidence of scoliosis in pinealectomized chicken. Spine (Phila Pa 1976) 2006;31(2):133–8.

30. Schmidt RE, Reavill DR, Phalen DN. Endocrine system. In: Schmidt RE, Phalen DN, editors. Pathology of pet and aviary birds. Ames (Iowa): Blackwell; 2003. p. 121.

31. Romagnano A. Pituitary adenoma in an Amazon Parrot. J Avian Med Surg 1995; 9(4):263–70.

32. Stiles J, Buyukmihci NC, Farver TB. Tonometry of normal eyes in raptors. Am J Vet Res 1994;55(4):477–9.

33. Roberson DW, Alosi JA, Cotanche DA. Direct transdifferentiation gives rise to the earliest new hair cells in regenerating avian auditory epithelium. J Neurosci Res 2004;78(4):461–71.

34. Muller M, Smolders JW. Responses of auditory nerve fibers innervating regenerated hair cells after local application of gentamicin at the round window of the cochlea in the pigeon. Hear Res 1999;131(1–2):153–69.

35. Cobb S. A note on the size of the avian olfactory bulb. Epilepsia 1960;1:394–402.

36. Steiger SS, Fidler AE, Valcu M. Avian olfactory receptor gene repertoires: evidence for a well-developed sense of smell in birds? Proc Biol Sci 2008; 275(1649):2309–17.

37. Balthazart J. Underestimated role of olfaction in avian reproduction? Behav Brain Res 2009;200(2):248–59.

38. Rothschild RM. Osteoarthritis is for the birds. Clin Rheumatol 2006;25(5):645–7.

39. Rothschild B, Panza R. Inverse relationship of osteoarthritis to weight: the bird lesson. Clin Exp Rheumatol 2006;24(2):218.

40. Norden CW. Lessons learned from animal models of osteomyelitis. Rev Infect Dis 1988;10(1):103–10.
41. Schmidt RE, Reavill DR, Phalen DN. The musculoskeletal system. In: Schmidt RE, Phalen DN, editors. Pathology of pet and aviary birds. Ames (Iowa): Blackwell; 2003. p. 149–63.
42. Stanford M. Calcium metabolism. In: Harrison GJ, Lightfoot TL, editors. Clinical avian medicine. Lake Worth (FL): Spix; 2006. p. 141–52.
43. Rhoden EL, Pereira-Lima J, Rhoden CR, et al. The role of colchicine in prevention of hepatic cirrhosis induced by carbon tetrachloride. Hepatogastroenterology 1999;46(26):1111–5.
44. Echols S. Evaluating and treating the kidneys. In: Harrison GJ, Lightfoot T, editors. Clinical avian medicine. Lake Worth (FL): Spix; 2006. p. 451–92.
45. McDonald DM. Nutritional considerations. In: Harrison GJ, Lightfoot TL, editors. Clinical avian medicine. Lake Worth (FL): Spix; 2006. p. 1125.
46. Dudas PL, Ryan MP, Eldon JB, et al. Transepithelial urate transport by avian renal proximal tubule epithelium in primary culture. J Exp Biol 2005;208(Pt 22): 4305–15.
47. Wideman RF, Chapman ME, Hamal KR, et al. An inadequate pulmonary vascular capacity and susceptibility to pulmonary arterial hypertension in broilers. Poult Sci 2007;86(5):984–98.
48. Tan X, Hu SH, Wang XL. Possible role of nitric oxide in the pathogenesis of pulmonary hypertension in broilers: a synopsis. Avian Pathol 2007;36(4):261–7.
49. Pees M, Krautwald-Junghanns M. Evaluating and treating the cardiovascular system. In: Harrison GJ, Lightfoot TL, editors. Clinical avian medicine. Lake Worth (FL): Spix; 2006. p. 379–94.
50. Blackburn R, Prashad D. The avian renal portal system: a model for studying nephrotoxicity of xenobiotics. Toxicol Lett 1990;53(1–2):219–21.
51. Schmidt RE, Reavill DR, Phalen DN. Cardiovascular system. In: Schmidt RE, Phalen DN, editors. Pathology of pet and aviary birds. Ames (Iowa): Blackwell; 2003. p. 51.
52. Krista LM, McDaniel GR, Mora EC, et al. Histological evaluation of the vascular system for the severity of atherosclerosis in hyper and hypotensive male and female turkeys: comparison between young and aged turkeys. Poult Sci 1987; 66(6):1033–44.
53. Bavelaar FJ, Beynen AC. Atherosclerosis in parrots. a review. Vet Q 2004;26(2): 50–60.
54. Dashti N, Kelley J, Thayer RH, et al. Concurrent inductions of avian hepatic lipogenesis, plasma lipids, and plasma apolipoprotein B by estrogen. J Lipid Res 1983;24(4):368–80.
55. Simone-Freilicher E. Use of isoxsuprine for treatment of clinical signs associated with presumptive atherosclerosis in a yellow-naped Amazon parrot (*Amazona ochrocephala auropalliata*). J Avian Med Surg 2007;21(3):215–9.
56. Sedacca CD, Campbell TW, Bright JM, et al. Chronic cor pulmonale secondary to pulmonary atherosclerosis in an African Grey parrot. J Am Vet Med Assoc 2009; 234(8):1055–9.
57. Shrubsole-Cockwill A, Wojnarowicz C, Parker D. Atherosclerosis and ischemic cardiomyopathy in a captive, adult red-tailed hawk (*Buteo jamaicensis*). Avian Dis 2008;52(3):537–9.
58. Mans C, Brown CJ. Radiographic evidence of atherosclerosis of the descending aorta in a grey-cheeked parakeet (*Brotogeris pyrrhopterus*). J Avian Med Surg 2007;21(1):56–62.

59. Bavelaar FJ, Beynen AC. Severity of atherosclerosis in parrots in relation to the intake of alpha-linolenic acid. Avian Dis 2003;47(3):566–77.
60. Phalen DN, Hays HB, Filippich LJ, et al. Heart failure in a macaw with atherosclerosis of the aorta and brachiocephalic arteries. J Am Vet Med Assoc 1996;209(8): 1435–40.
61. Muwalla MM, Abuirmeileh NM. Suppression of avian hepatic cholesterogenesis by dietary ginseng. J Nutr Biochem 1990;1(10):518–21.
62. Acierno MJ, da Cunha A, Smith J, et al. Agreement between direct and indirect blood pressure measurements obtained from anesthetized Hispaniolan Amazon parrots. J Am Vet Med Assoc 2008;233(10):1587–90.
63. Rembert MS, Smith JA, Strickland KN, et al. Intermittent bradyarrhythmia in a Hispaniolan Amazon parrot (Amazona ventralis). J Avian Med Surg 2008;22(1): 31–40.
64. Schmidt RE, Reavill DR, Phalen DN. Reproductive System. In: Schmidt RE, Reavill DR, Phalen DN, editors. Pathology of caged and aviary birds. Ames (Iowa): Blackwell; 2003. p. 109–20.
65. Bentley GE, Ubuka T, McGuire NL, et al. Gonadotropin-inhibitory hormone and its receptor in the avian reproductive system. Gen Comp Endocrinol 2008;156(1): 34–43.
66. Schmidt R, Lightfoot TL. Integument. In: Harrison GJ, Lightfoot TL, editors. Clinical avian medicine. Lake Worth (FL): Spix; 2006. p. 395–409.
67. Lightfoot TL. Clinical avian neoplasia and oncology. In: Harrison GJ, Lightfoot TL, editors. Clinical avian medicine. Lake Worth (FL): Spix publishing; 2006. p. 560–6.
68. Tully TN. Liposarcomas in a monk parakeet (Myiopsitta monachus). J Assoc Avian Vet 1994;8(3):120–4.
69. Schmidt RE, Reavill DR, Phalen DN. Integumentary system. In: Schmidt RE, Reavill DR, Phalen DN, editors. Pathology of caged and aviary birds. Ames (Iowa): Blackwell; 2003. p. 21.
70. Suedmeyer W. Attempted photodynamic therapy of squamous cell carcinoma in the casque of a great hornbill (Buceros bicornis). J Avian Med Surg 2001;15(1): 44–9.
71. Rosenthal K. A report of photodynamic therapy for squamous cell carcinoma in a cockatiel. In: RK, editor. Proc ann conf AAV; 2001. p. 175–6.
72. MacWhirter P. Use of carboplatin in the treatment of renal adenocarcinoma in a budgerigar. Exotic DVM 2002;4(2):11–2.
73. Watson CL. Primary appendicular bone tumors in dogs. Compend Contin Educ Pract Vet 2002;24(2):128–38.
74. Zantopp DA. Treatment of bile duct carcinoma in birds with carboplatin. Exotic DVM 2000;2(3):76–8.
75. Filippich L. Intravenous cisplatin administration in sulphur-crested cockatoos (Cacatua galerita) clinical and pathologic observations. J Avian Med Surg 2001;15(1):23–30.
76. Filippich LJ, Charles BG, Sutton RH, et al. Carboplatin administration in sulphur-crested cockatoos (Cacatua galerita): clinical observations. J Avian Med Surg 2005;19(2):92–7.
77. Crosta L, Gerlach H, Bürkle M, et al. Physiology, diagnosis, and diseases of the avian reproductive tract. Veterinary Clin North Am Exot Anim Pract 2003;6(1): 57–83.
78. Urick ME, Giles JR, Johnson PA. Dietary aspirin decreases the stage of ovarian cancer in the hen. Gynecol Oncol 2009;112(1):166–70.

79. Weniger JP, Samsel J. Tamoxifen and ovarian differentiation in birds. Arch Anat Microsc Morphol Exp 1985;74(1):50–1.
80. Mani C, Pearce R, Parkinson A, et al. Involvement of cytochrome P4503A in catalysis of tamoxifen activation and covalent binding to rat and human liver microsomes. Carcinogenesis 1994;15(12):2715–20.
81. Lupu CA. Evaluation of side effects of tamoxifen in budgerigars (*Melopsittacus undulatus*). J Avian Med Surg 2000;14(4):237–42.
82. Schmidt RE, Reavill DR, Phalen DN. Gastrointestinal system and pancreas. In: Schmidt RE, Reavill DR, Phalen DN, editors. Pathology of pet and aviary birds. Ames (Iowa): Blackwell; 2003. p. 41–65.
83. Hillyer EV, Moroff S, Hoefer H, et al. Bile duct carcinoma in two out of ten Amazon parrots with cloacal papillomas. J Assoc Avian Vet 1999;5(2):91–5.
84. Phalen DN. Implication of viruses in clinical disorders. In: Harrison GJ, Lightfoot TL, editors. Clinical avian medicine. Lake Worth (FL): Spix; 2006. p. 721–45.
85. Schmidt RE, Reavill DR, Phalen DN. Hemopoetic and lymphatic systems. In: Schmidt RE, Reavill DR, Phalen DN, editors. Pathology of caged and aviary birds. Ames (Iowa): Blackwell; 2006. p. 102–31.
86. Garner MM. A retrospective study of case submissions to a specialty diagnostic service. In: Harrison GJ, Lightfoot TL, editors. Clinical avian medicine. Lake Worth (FL): Spix; 2006. p. 566–73.
87. Cambell TW. Carcinoma of the ventriculus with metastasis to the lungs in a sulphur-crested cockatoo (*Cacatua galerita*). J Avian Med Surg 1999;13(4):265–8.
88. Jones MP, Orosz S. Pulmonary carcinoma with metastases in a moluccan cockatoo (*Cacatua moluccensis*). J Avian Med Surg 2001;15(2):107–13.

The Aging Raptor

Tim Tristan, DVM

KEYWORDS

• Raptor • Bird of prey • Age • Geriatric

Birds of prey have been used in various manners by humans, worldwide, for centuries. Despite this fact, the information available in the literature on geriatric raptors is sparse, anecdotal, and written in various languages and journals that may not be easily accessible. Veterinarians beginning a career with raptors have a daunting task ahead of them. Becoming familiar with species commonly encountered, their natural history, husbandry requirements, dietary needs, and basic disease conditions is the foundation of raptor medicine. These fundamentals will allow the veterinarian to more correctly identify symptoms that may reflect geriatric conditions and aid in age determination of raptors on presentation. The goal of this article is to expose the reader to the numerous aspects that may affect raptor survival, longevity, and health. In addition, the most frequently seen geriatric disease conditions are reviewed.

RAPTORS AND THEIR USE BY HUMANS
Falconry

According to some experts, the origins of falconry date back to 4000 to 6000 BC in the steppes of Mongolia. Other historians have found records identifying birds of prey being used in Iran over 8,000 to 10,000 years ago. Falconry became well established in Asia and the Middle East by 2000 BC, and soon after migrated to Europe. Birds of prey were a status symbol and the sport of royalty from the sixth century through the Middle Ages. In the 1600s in England, the Laws of Ownership were used to allow citizens of various social rank to fly certain birds of prey. Popularity in Europe began to decrease in the 1800s because of the increased use of firearms, decline of the aristocracy, and land development for agriculture. Resurgence was not seen again until the 1920s and 1930s.

In North America, falconry dates back to the early 1500s, when the Aztecs used trained hawks. The first documentation of falconry in the United States was in New England in 1622. The first falconry association established in the United States was the Falconer's Association of North America in 1940, but it was disbanded during World War II. Since that time, the North American Falconry Association (NAFA) was formed in 1961 and currently has more than 2000 members.

As expected, medical conditions and treatments have been identified and used since the early days of falconry. Early writings of European falconers of the thirteenth

VCA Oso Creek Animal Hospital, 7713 South Staples, Corpus Christi, TX 78413, USA
E-mail address: exoticvet@yahoo.com

Vet Clin Exot Anim 13 (2010) 51–84
doi:10.1016/j.cvex.2009.10.001   **vetexotic.theclinics.com**
1094-9194/10/$ – see front matter © 2010 Elsevier Inc. All rights reserved.

to the nineteenth centuries describe many of the disease conditions encountered today.[1] Falconry husbandry techniques have historically been one of the primary modalities used to care for and treat birds of prey. Fortunately, advancement of veterinary care for falconry birds has resulted in falconers more frequently turning to veterinarians for care and treatment of their birds. Institutions such as the Abu Dhabi Research Hospital have led the way for specialized veterinary care for falconry birds.[2]

Zoologic Institutions

Displaying raptors is commonplace in most zoologic facilities exhibiting birds. Institutions not only exhibit birds of prey but also have demonstrations, interactive programs, and shows that allow the public to view these birds performing many of their natural behaviors. The combination of educating while entertaining is a powerful tool that is used by most institutions to raise awareness for target species. In addition, many zoos are involved in conservation efforts locally and internationally to increase public awareness and help secure sustainability of sensitive species through efforts ranging from fundraising to captive breeding. One unique aspect of raptors housed in captivity is the absence of environmental pressures, which results in increased life expectancy when compared with their wild counterparts. The overall increase in the number of zoos, birds housed at these institutions, and successful conservation projects has resulted in a greater need for veterinary care for these specialized birds.

Due to the increased longevity of raptors kept in zoologic collections, veterinarians have had the opportunity and ability to observe, document, diagnose, and treat various conditions, both common and uncommon. The advent of advanced diagnostic testing, including molecular techniques and diagnostic imaging, has also aided in the improvement of raptor medicine. Furthermore, development of new diagnostics and therapies has resulted in increased life expectancy of many individuals who in the past would have gone undiagnosed or untreated. The results of conservation efforts by zoologic facilities, biologists, and veterinarians can be seen with species such as the bald eagle, California condor, peregrine falcon, Aplomado falcon, and many others around the world.

Wildlife

Significant research and conservation efforts have been performed by scientists, biologists, ornithologists, naturalists, and veterinarians in the area of the natural history and medicine of wild raptors. Investigation into the natural history of these birds has expanded the basic knowledge of many species and has allowed a better understanding of many unfamiliar aspects of these birds, including migratory routes, hunting techniques, and reproduction. Molecular testing has been used to evaluate genetic diversity and identify gender prior to hatching. Naturalists are a key motivating and influential component to evaluation of wildlife. Events such as the Christmas Bird Count, Whooping Crane Festival, Florida Keys Raptor Migration Project, and others are prime examples of community involvement in the preservation and protection of wildlife. Whereas many of these events are casual, others are strictly scientific and are important indicators of the wild populations, and may provide the first indications of serious impacts and trends on wildlife.

The encroachment of human development into naive areas inhabited by raptors has resulted in an increased number of injuries and mortality. The increased impact on wildlife has motivated individuals and organizations to establish wildlife rescue and rehabilitation facilities to care for these birds. National and international organizations such as IWRC (International Wildlife Rehabilitation Counsel) and NWRA (National Wildlife Rehabilitators Association) have also been formed to collectively disseminate knowledge with regard to rescuing, rehabilitating, and releasing birds as well as educating the public. Most large metropolitan cities have raptor rescue organizations that play a key role in rehabilitation. The information gathered from rehabilitation facilities and veterinarians has been an invaluable resource for expanding the practice of raptor medicine and surgery.

Divisions of Raptors

The distinction between falconry birds, zoo exhibit birds, and wildlife are identified to make the clinician aware that these divisions may alter the definition of what is considered a "geriatric" raptor. Even though there are morphologic characteristics in various raptor species that enable them to be identified as hatchlings, juveniles, sub-adults, and adults, determining the age of an adult raptor with an unknown history is difficult if not impossible.

Age Determination in Raptors

Identifying the correct age of raptors is fraught with endless variables that must be taken into consideration. Young raptors may be identified by behavioral and morphologic characteristics that employ both subjective and objective observations.[3–9] Young raptors may be recognized over the first few years of life by their plumage (**Figs. 1–6**). Some raptor species maintain their juvenile plumage for 1 to 2 years, whereas other species, such as the bald eagle, may maintain their juvenile plumage for up to 4 to 5 years. Behavioral aspects may also indicate that an individual is young, even though it may have adult plumage. Juvenile birds often are presented to rehabilitation facilities due to traumatic injuries while hunting. Other individuals may be emaciated and weak due to their lack of hunting experience soon after fledging.

Adult raptors are significantly more difficult to age. Behavioral and morphologic characteristics are of little aid except to differentiate adults from the juveniles. The most helpful tool used to determine age of raptors is record keeping. Documentation by falconers, scientists, naturalists, and veterinarians is often the only way to determine their age. The use of radio telemetry, leg bands, microchips, and medical records have also been incorporated in studying these birds.[10–12] Organizations such as Hawk Watch International are important contributors to increasing the knowledge base for raptor aging and longevity.

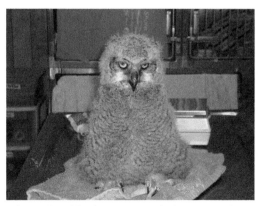

Fig. 1. Juvenile great horned owl (*Bubo virginianus*). (*Courtesy of* Tim Tristan, DVM.)

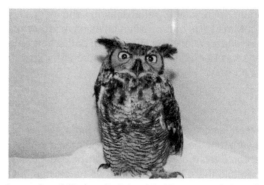

Fig. 2. Adult great horned owl (*Bubo virginianus*). (*Courtesy of* Tim Tristan, DVM.)

Aging raptors for all intensive purposes is an inexact science unless meticulous record keeping has been performed or is available. Therefore, identifying the geriatric raptor by the veterinarian requires a compilation of the information already stated in addition to the history, signalment, symptoms, and clinical signs.

Morbidity, Mortality, and Life Expectancy

One approach to recognizing geriatric raptors is identifying morbidity and mortality events and their frequency, impact, and effect on raptor populations. These variables have a direct correlation with the life expectancy of wild raptors. The most well-documented morbidity and mortality reports in the literature involve wild populations of birds of prey. Record life spans are listed in **Table 1**.

Morbidity and mortality reports can be classified into 2 categories, human influence and environmental impact. Human influence affects birds of prey both directly and indirectly. The majority of mortality events in raptors are due to traumatic injuries.[17–23] Traumatic injuries may be the result of vehicular impact, collision with buildings, unspecified impact injuries, or gunshot wounds.[17,21,22,24–28]

Indirect impacts by humans may also be seen in the form of toxicoses and land development for human use.[29] The most well-publicized toxins affecting birds of prey are dichlorodiphenyltrichloroethane (DDT) and lead. DDT resulted in a worldwide decrease in raptor populations. Since that time, DDT has been banned in most developed countries.[30] Lead has also been identified as having a significant effect on raptor

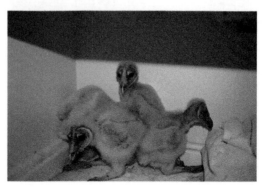

Fig. 3. Juvenile barn owls (*Tyto alba*). (*Courtesy of* Tim Tristan, DVM.)

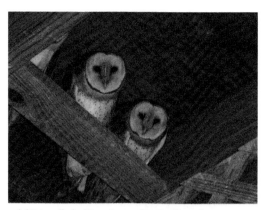

Fig. 4. Adult barn owl (*Tyto alba*). (*Courtesy of* Kelly Shutt.)

populations. Lead exposure is generally due to ingestion of prey items containing lead shot, fishing sinkers, or high tissue-lead concentrations.[31–33] The toxic side effects of lead have resulted in the ban of lead shot in North American wetlands and other places around the world. Non-lead alternatives such as steel, tungsten-nickel-iron, and bismuth-tin are now being used. There are numerous other toxins that are being investigated such as mercury, cadmium, chromium, diclofenac, famphur, carbofuran, fensulfothion, second-generation anticoagulant rodenticides, and numerous organophosphates/carbamates and organochlorines.[34–44] Toxic compounds remain a serious threat to wild raptor populations.

Human development in previously unpopulated areas results in more encounters with wildlife, including raptors and their food sources. This encroachment often results in displacement of birds from their native hunting grounds and a decrease in their home range. Hakkarainen and colleagues[45] discovered that the annual survival of Tengmalm's owl was dependent on cover of old coniferous forests, and suggested that changes in habitat created by agriculture and forestry development may reduce adult survivability. Similar reports have prompted conservation efforts that also ensure preservation of habitat for raptor species. Electrocution from power lines and trauma from collisions with wind power generators have also been identified as causes of

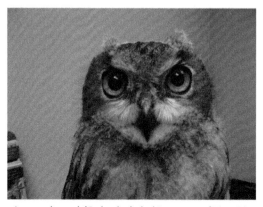

Fig. 5. Juvenile Eurasian eagle owl (*Bubo bubo*). (*Courtesy of* Tim Tristan, DVM.)

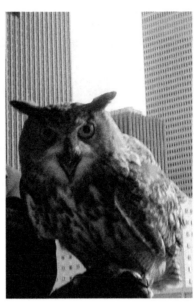

Fig. 6. Adult Eurasian eagle owl (*Bubo bubo*). (*Courtesy of* Patty Shoemaker Downtown Aquarium, Houston, TX.)

mortality in raptors (**Figs. 7** and **8**).[17,21,24,25,46] The increase in the number of wind power generators over the coming years may have a significant impact in raptor populations.

Environmental factors may also affect the survivability and longevity of raptors. Natural disasters such as forest fires, hurricanes, tornados, and extreme weather events (ie, winter freezes), may significantly impact wild populations. Two extreme winters in Switzerland resulted in major population declines in barn owls.[47] Sarasola and colleagues[48] reported 113 Swainson's hawks and 45 birds of 11 other species that were found dead as a result of a single hailstorm in the Argentina Pampas. The event does not seem to be an isolated incident, as landowners have provided further evidence of past hailstorms with similar results.

Morbidity and mortality due to natural causes may be the result of predation, intraspecific conflict, orphaned young, starvation, infection, and metabolic, neoplastic, and degenerative diseases.[49] Heckel and colleagues[50] documented 3 cases of suspected fatal snakebite inflicted on 2 juvenile red-tailed hawks and one adult Cooper's hawk. Infectious causes of mortality may include bacterial, fungal, viral infections, and parasitism.[51–53] The most recent viral infection affecting wild raptor populations in North America is the West Nile virus.[54–57] Other viral infections that have been identified in raptors include Columbid herpesvirus-1 in 2 Cooper's hawks and falcon adenovirus in an American kestrel (*Falco sparverius*).[58,59] Further medical conditions are covered later in the article.

The age of some falconry birds may be known, often due to the fact that they were caught while in juvenile plumage or they were hatched by a falconer or aviculturist. Other birds used by falconers are of unknown age, and estimations must be made. In addition, many birds are used for hunting for only one season and subsequently released. Morbidity and mortality reports of falconry birds are sparse to nonexistent. Two reports in the literature revealed trauma as the primary cause of death in trained

Table 1
Longevity records of raptors (wild, falconry, and zoo birds)

Common Name	Scientific Name	Record Life Span	References
Turkey vulture	Cathartes arua	20 y	[13]
Eurasian black vulture	Aegypius monachus	39 y	[13]
White-backed vulture	Gyps africanus	19 y	[13]
Egyptian vulture	Neophron percnopterus	37 y	[13]
Black vulture	Coragyps atratus	25 y 6 mo	[14]
King vulture	Sarcoramphus papa	>40 y	Flanagan J, personal communication, 2009
Bearded vulture	Gypaetus barbatus	>40 y	[15]
Andean condor	Vultur gryphus	75 y	[13]
California condor	Gymnogyps californianus	45 y	[13]
Black-shouldered kite	Elanus caeruleus	6 y	[13]
Square-tailed kite	Lophoictinia isura	17 y	[13]
Black kite	Milvus migrans	24 y	[13]
White-tailed kite	Elanus leucurus	5 y 11 mo	[14]
Mississippi kite	Ictinia mississippiensis	11 y 2 mo	[14]
Snail kite	Rostrhamus sociabilis	17 y	[13]
Red kite	Milvus milvus	38 y	[15]
Swamp harrier	Circus aeruginosus	20 y	[13]
Pallid harrier	Circus macrourus	13 y	[13]
Montagu's harrier	Circus pygargus	16 y	[13]
Northern harrier	Circus cyaneus	16 y 5 mo	[14]
Sharp-shinned hawk	Accipiter striatus	19 y 11 mo	[14]
Cooper's hawk	Accipiter cooperii	20 y 4 mo	[14]
Northern goshawk	Accipiter gentilis	>28 y	[14]
Harris' hawk	Parabuteo unicinctus	25 y	[13]
Red-tailed hawk	Buteo jamaicensis	28 y 10 mo	[14]
Common buzzard	Buteo Buteo	24 y	[14]
Red-shouldered hawk	Buteo lineatus	19 y 11 mo	[14]
Swainson's hawk	Buteo swainsonii	24 y 1 mo	[14]
Broad-winged hawk	Buteo platypterus	18 y	[13]
Rough-legged hawk	Buteo lagopus	18 y	[13]
Ferruginous hawk	Buteo regalis	23 y 8 mo	[14]
Hawaiian hawk	Buteo solitarius	17 y	[13]
Common black hawk	Buteogallus anthracinus	13 y	[13]
Golden eagle	Aquila chrysaetos	>48 y	[15]
Bald eagle	Haliaeetus leucocephalus	31 y 4 mo	[14]
White-tailed sea eagle	Haliaeetus albicilla	95 y	[15]
Spanish imperial eagle	Aquila adalberti	44 y 5 mo	[13]
Wedge-tailed eagle	Aquila audax	40 y	[13]
Eastern imperial eagle	Aquila heliaca	56 y	[13]
Steppe eagle	Aquila nipalensis	41 y	[13]
Lesser spotted eagle	Aquila pomarina	26 y	[13]
Tawny eagle	Aquila rapax	40 y	[13]
Short-toed eagle	Circaetus gallicus	17 y	[13]

(continued on next page)

	Table 1 (continued)		
Common Name	**Scientific Name**	**Record Life Span**	**References**
Chilean eagle	*Geranoaetus melanoleucus*	42 y	13
Sea eagle	*Gypohierax angolensis*	27 y	13
Harpy eagle	*Harpia harpyja*	16 y	13
New Guinea eagle	*Harpyopsis novaeguineae*	30 y	13
Bonelli's eagle	*Hieraaetus fasciatus*	20 y	13
Little eagle	*Hieraaetus morphnoides*	10 y	13
Philippine eagle	*Pithecophaga jefferyi*	41 y	13
Eurasian eagle-owl	*Bubo bubo*	68 y	13
Saker falcon	*Falco cherrug*	29 y	15
Brown falcon	*Falco berigora*	16 y	13
Eleonora's falcon	*Falco eleonorae*	11 y	13
Red-footed falcon	*Falco vespertinus*	13 y	13
Gyrfalcon	*Falco rusticolus*	13 y 6 mo	14
Mauritius kestrel	*Falco punctatus*	10 y 10 d	16
Eurasian kestrel	*Falco tinnunculus*	23 y	13
American kestrel	*Falco sparverius*	17 y	13
Lesser kestrel	*Falco naumanni*	10 y	13
Prairie falcon	*Falco mexicanus*	17 y 3 mo	14
Peregrine falcon	*Falco peregrinus*	25 y	13
Merlin	*Falco columbarius*	12 y	15
Aplomado falcon	*Falco femoralis*	12 y	13
Crested caracara	*Caracara cheriway*	25 y 8 mo	13
Southern caracara	*Caracara plancus*	37 y 6 mo	13
Osprey	*Pandion haliaetus*	26 y 2 mo	14
Bateleur	*Terathopius ecaudatus*	>55 y	15
Barn owl	*Tyto alba*	28 y	Flanagan J, personal communication, 2009
Long-eared owl	*Asio otus*	27 y	13
Short-eared owl	*Asio flammeus*	21 y 5 mo	14
Barred owl	*Strix varia*	18 y 2 mo	14
Spotted owl	*Strix occidentalis*	21 y	14
Great gray owl	*Strix nebulosa*	12 y 9 mo	14
Boreal owl	*Aegolius funereus*	15 y	13
Northern saw-whet owl	*Aegolius acadicus*	17 y	13
Eastern screech owl	*Otus asio*	20 y	14
Western screech owl	*Otus kennicottii*	19 y	13
Flammulated owl	*Otus flammeolus*	7 y	14
Great horned owl	*Bubo virginianus*	29 y	14
Snowy owl	*Nyctea scandiaca*	28 y	13
Burrowing owl	*Athene cunicularis*	11 y	13
Little owl	*Athene noctua*	9 y	13
Eurasian pygmy owl	*Glaucidium passerinum*	6 y	13
Eurasian scops-owl	*Otus scops*	6 y	13
Elf owl	*Micrathene whitneyi*	14 y	13

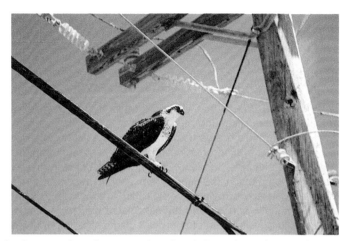

Fig. 7. Birds of prey, such as this osprey (*Pandion haliaetus*), are frequently seen perched on power lines while hunting for prey. (*Courtesy of* Tim Tristan, DVM.)

raptors.[60,61] One report involved the British Falconry Club (BFC) where 197 trained raptors were followed over a 6-year period and 76 (38.5%) deaths were recorded. Twenty-four (12.1%) birds died as a result of trauma. Anecdotal reports also support that a common cause of raptor mortality is trauma, whereas others report infectious disease, ophthalmic disease, and organ failure as being more common.

Probably the best documentation of geriatric raptors is by zoologic institutions and educational facilities. These birds may have been acquired through breeding programs, conservation projects, and wildlife rehabilitation centers. Many birds used for educational programs or exhibits originate from rehabilitation facilities where it has been determined the animal is unfit for release. Other projects, such as the California Condor Conservation project, are an integral part of zoo and wildlife conservation efforts in expanding the knowledge base of the many aspects of their care. Rehabilitation facilities frequently use nonreleasable individuals as animal ambassadors to educate the public on the pressures inflicted by humans on birds of prey.

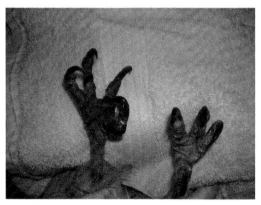

Fig. 8. A red tailed hawk (*Buteo jamaicensis*) found near an electrical transformer had severe burns on the talons leading to a diagnosis of electrocution. (*Courtesy of* Tim Tristan, DVM.)

When compared with other methods of evaluating morbidity and mortality reports of geriatric birds, zoo and educational birds are the most significant resource available.

DISEASE CONDITIONS
Musculoskeletal Diseases (Degenerative Joint Disease and Osteoarthritis)

Musculoskeletal changes due to age are most often related to osteoarthritis and degenerative joint diseases. Although these terms may be interchanged frequently, they are distinct. Osteoarthritis is a pathologic change of a diarthrodial synovial articulation, including the deterioration of articular cartilage, osteophyte formation, bone remodeling, soft tissue changes, and low-grade nonpurulent inflammation. Degenerative joint disease, in comparison, is a general term used to describe any degenerative change in synovial cartilaginous or fibrous articulation in the skeleton. The increase in life expectancy in domestic animals and the associated geriatric conditions such as arthritis has resulted in development of improved diagnostics and treatment modalities for these patients. The information gained from domestic species has allowed for a better understanding of these conditions in avian species, although much work remains to be done.

Few reports in the literature discuss osteoarthritis or degenerative joint diseases in birds as it relates to age. Disease conditions such as gout, bacterial and fungal osteomyelitis, and trauma-related injures comprise the majority of bone- and joint-related reports. Rothschild and Panza[62] examined museum specimens of 2243 free-ranging hawks and determined that 3% had osteoarthritis, all localized to the ankle. In addition, there was not enough evidence to correlate age with the development of osteoarthritis. Despite this fact, geriatric birds seen by veterinarians frequently present with bone- and joint-related disease conditions. Cooper[63] describes a condition seen in older raptors resembling rheumatoid arthritis in which one or both legs become stiff and the bird is unable to stand. The patients' symptoms may resolve but often reoccur with intermittent signs of collapse. A cardiovascular component to the condition has been hypothesized. Many raptors examined by veterinarians have preexisting medical conditions that predispose them to arthritis. Previous traumatic injuries are the most common cause of development of arthritis in patients seen by the author. Wing injuries involving the humerus, radius, ulna, and carpus have all been associated with development of osteoarthritis and degenerative joint disease. Osteoarthritis also occurs in the long bones of the legs, but is less frequently observed in comparison with the wing. Fractures that are near the joints appear to result in the most severe cases of degenerative joint disease and osteoarthritis. The contradiction in reports of osteoarthritis in wild caught birds as opposed to that described anecdotally by veterinarians may be due to the status of the birds (ie, wild vs captive). Wild birds that are presented to rehabilitation facilities rarely have chronic bone or joint disease. The limited number of raptors presented to rehabilitation facilities with chronic joint injuries is likely due to their decreased ability to effectively hunt and sustain their caloric needs in the wild.

Falconry birds with osteoarthritis and degenerative joint disease of the shoulder, elbow, carpus, stifle, and tarsus are seen occasionally. The most frequent diagnosis of arthritis in falconry birds made by the author is related to the elbow and tarsus. Historical reports of trauma and bumblefoot related injuries seem to be predisposing factors affecting the development of osteoarthritis in these 2 areas. Raptors in zoologic collections seen with osteoarthritis and degenerative joint disease are becoming more frequent due to the increased longevity and extensive veterinary care these birds receive. In the author's experience, arthritis in these individuals is most frequently located in the stifle and tarsus; this is likely due to lack of conditioning or obesity.

Arthritis is usually is suspected due to clinical signs. Arthritis related to the legs may result in shifting leg lameness, development of bumblefoot, joint and leg swelling, edema, uncoordinated movements, curling of the foot, and decreased range of motion. Arthritis related to the wings may also result in many of the same conditions, including wing drooping or inability to place the wing in full extension or flexion. Raptors that are part of a show or program will frequently exhibit behavioral cues that indicate there may be a problem. Decreased activity level, inability to capture and hold prey, failure to meet criteria for specific behaviors, and inappetence may all be observed by falconers, keepers, and trainers as well as veterinarians.

A thorough physical examination should begin with visual examination of the patient before the "hands on" examination. Most birds of prey, like many other avian species, will appear normal on first glance. Given time, once the birds become more comfortable with their surroundings and presence of onlookers, clinical signs may be noted. Only when the bird has been fully evaluated visually should it be captured for the physical examination. Many veterinarians perform a physical examination and then perform a more in-depth orthopedic examination to evaluate bone and joint conditions. The orthopedic examination is conducted on the legs and wings, starting distally and working toward the most proximal joint. Each joint is manipulated in flexion and extension to evaluate for crepitus, decreased range of motion, or other abnormalities. Care must be taken by the examiner when evaluating the feet as injury may occur if taloned by the patient. On completion of the physical examination, diagnostics may be pursued.

The primary diagnostic used to evaluate for osteoarthritis and degenerative joint disease is radiography. The advent of digital radiography has revolutionized diagnostic imaging for evaluating birds, including raptors. Ultrasound, computed tomography, and magnetic resonance imaging have also been used to further evaluate patients. Once the region of arthritis has been identified, a thorough diagnostic workup should be performed to identify the possible cause. Infectious, inflammatory, traumatic, neoplastic, nutritional, metabolic, and other differentials should be excluded before a final diagnosis of a degenerative joint or bone condition is definitively diagnosed.

Treatment of osteoarthritis should be addressed using a multimodal approach. First, identification of the arthritic location and the classification of the joint or bone should be performed. The classification of the joint (ie, fibrous, cartilaginous, synovial) may dictate which treatments may be most advantageous for the patient. In addition, husbandry conditions may need to be modified to improve the outcome.

Husbandry changes may include perch selection, exhibit location, activities performed, and environmental exposure. Obesity may complicate osteoarthritis and exacerbate the condition. For this reason, a raptor's weight should be monitored frequently, if not daily, to allow adjustments when needed. Weight management not only decreases the load the joints must carry but also prevents other conditions such as hepatic lipidosis. Osteoarthritis in the legs and feet frequently causes redistribution of weight onto the less affected foot, and may result in bumblefoot. Multiple perches of various sizes with appropriate cover (ie, artificial turf) should be used to aid in prevention of foot lesions caused by inappropriate weight distribution (**Fig. 9**). Birds on exhibit may select perches that are inappropriate for their needs to avoid close association with the public or staff. Thought should be given to the types of materials being used and the location in which they are being placed. Individuals that fly in shows or hunt may have to decrease the frequency with which they perform these tasks to prevent further damage or more serious life-threatening injuries. Removal from shows or hunting should be done in a gradual manner to prevent

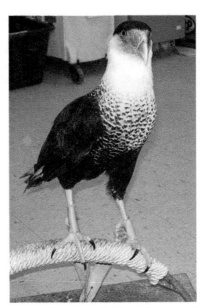

Fig. 9. Osteoarthritis is seen more frequently in birds of prey such as this Southern Caracara (*Caracara plancus*) due to their increased longevity in captivity. Visualizing subtle clinical signs requires visual observation of the patient before restraint and "hands on" exam. (*Courtesy of* Tim Tristan, DVM.)

disease conditions such as avascular necrosis of the third digit, as seen in some raptors in the Middle East after the hunting season.[64] These determinations are made on a case by case basis and criteria for these decisions depend on the severity of the arthritis, other disease conditions, and experience of the falconer, keepers, or trainers. The stress of performing or being on exhibit for extended periods of time are factors that may be manipulated for some geriatric raptors to improve their well-being.

Pharmaceutical therapy is the most common and beneficial tool used by veterinarians to treat osteoarthritis. Multiple drugs are being used, with marked success, in many domestic and avian species. Nonsteroidal anti-inflammatory drugs (NSAIDS) are probably the most frequently used drugs, prescribed for their anti-inflammatory and analgesic properties in birds.[65–71] Unfortunately, limited pharmacokinetic data exist for their use in avian species. In domestic species that have been studied more extensively, patients are monitored for side effects related to liver function, renal function, and gastrointestinal erosions. In these species, a standard hematology and chemistry profile is performed before initiating therapy, and periodically thereafter. The same protocol is recommended in birds before starting NSAID therapy. If renal, hepatic, or gastrointestinal conditions are identified before starting NSAIDS, consideration must be given to the benefit versus risk. Many of these drugs (aspirin, ketoprofen, ibuprofen, flunixin meglumine, phenylbutazone) have fallen out of favor due to toxic side effects seen in birds, including renal failure, prolonged clotting times, and gastrointestinal ulceration.[72] At present, the 2 most frequently used NSAIDS used in avian species are carprofen (Rimadyl) and meloxicam (Metacam). Both drugs have shown adequate analgesia in osteoarthritis as well as other painful conditions, and minimal side effects compared with their predecessors. Other NSAIDS such as celecoxib are being used in psittacines, but their use in raptors has not yet been evaluated.[73]

Opioids, although used commonly in domestic animals such as dogs and cats, have had limited use in avian species. Part of the reason is a lack of published data on opiate receptors and their distribution and function in avian species. There is increasing debate over the roles of κ, μ, and δ receptors and their response to specific opiates. Morphine, butorphanol, buprenorphine, fentanyl, and codeine have all been investigated for their use in birds, but few have been evaluated for their use in raptors.[72,74–85] Opioids are most often used for presurgical administration in birds, but are rarely used long term in any species because of potential side effects including cardiac and respiratory depression, sedation, euphoria, inappetence, and constipation.

Tramadol is used for pain control in several different species due to its affinity for the μ receptor, yet it is not classified as an opioid. Tramadol is thought to provide analgesia by acting on opioid, serotonin, and norepinephrine pathways.[86] Tramadol is frequently used for chronic pain in other species, and is thought to work synergistically with NSAIDS. A study performed by Souza and colleagues[87] evaluated 6 bald eagles administered tramadol intravenously and orally to determine plasma concentrations over time.[87] The author has used tramadol, 1 to 4 mg/kg, in raptors and psittacines, with promising results. In 2 cases of osteoarthritis in red-tailed hawks (*Buteo jamaicensis*) older than 20 years, positive results were noted by trainers and staff, with no evidence of side effects. Further investigations need to be performed to evaluate the analgesic properties of tramadol in raptors.

Nutraceuticals are often used as part of the treatment protocol for many species with osteoarthritis. Products such as Cosequin, Adequan, and others contain glucosamine, chondroitin sulfate, and Omega-3 fatty acids. These products are intended to help rebuild the cartilage that has broken down over time and repair damage that has been done. Although there are few reports in the literature, the author has seen positive results with Cosequin administered orally to several avian species including raptors.[88]

Tricyclic antidepressants including amitriptyline, clomipramine, and imipramine provide relief to individuals with chronic neuropathic pain, and are thought to alter the actions of serotonin and norepinephrine both centrally and peripherally.[89] The majority of the reports related to birds in the literature are in reference to feather picking and self-mutilating psittacines. The use of tricyclic antidepressants in raptors remains to be seen. Conditions such as self-mutilation in Harris hawks may also benefit from this class of drug.[90,91]

The anticonvulsant gabapentin is clinically effective in relieving some types of chronic pain in people, and has been used in dogs and cats, yet the mechanism of action is unclear. Side effects seen in cats include ataxia and sedation. One report of gabapentin use in birds reported a dose of 10 mg/kg given twice a day by mouth in a little corella.[92] A second case of a Senegal parrot (*Poicephalus senegalus*) with leg twitching and foot mutilation caused by neuralgia reported the use of gabapentin at a dose of 3 mg/kg every 24 hours by mouth to be effective.[93] To the author's knowledge there are no reports of gabapentin use in raptors.

Physical therapy, including passive range of motion and techniques used by falconers for conditioning, can aid in treatment of osteoarthritis and result in an improved quality of life. Rehabilitation and physical therapy are discussed in a later section.

Neoplasia

Neoplastic disease conditions have been reported in the literature with increased frequency as the life span of birds has steadily increased. Neoplastic conditions reported in raptors are listed in **Table 2**. Diagnosis of neoplasia is dependent on history and physical examination findings, but may also require advanced diagnostic techniques. Radiography, computed tomography, ultrasonography, cytology, and histopathology may each be crucial in the definitive diagnosis of neoplasia.

Treatment of neoplastic disease conditions depends on the type, location, expected response to therapy, and condition of the patient. Once these variables have been determined, a palliative, moderate, or aggressive course of therapy should be chosen. Therapy may include surgical excision, cryotherapy, chemotherapy, photodynamic therapy, radiation therapy, or any combination of these. Most neoplastic tumors in raptors reported in the literature have been surgically excised.[94] Chemotherapy agents including prednisolone, doxorubicin, cisplatin, carboplatin, chlorambucil, cyclophosphamide, vincristine, and α-interferon have all been used in the treatment of specific neoplastic conditions in other orders of birds, primarily psittacines.[98–105] Radiation therapy was performed in a golden eagle (*Aquila chrysaetos*) with squamous cell carcinoma.[106–108] Although neoplastic conditions may occur in raptors at any age, they primarily occur in older geriatric raptors.

Cardiovascular Disease

Cardiovascular disease in avian species has recently received more attention in the veterinary literature, yet the information available is still limited. In addition, most reports of cardiovascular disease involve psittacines, and those in raptors are primarily diagnosed post mortem. Finding cardiovascular disease on postmortem examination also leaves the question of whether the cardiovascular disease was the primary cause of death, a contributory cause of death, or an incidental finding. A combination of history, physical examination, clinical signs, and diagnostic testing may need to be used to formulate a diagnosis and illuminate the affects associated with cardiovascular disease in raptors.

The physical examination should begin with a visual assessment of the bird in its enclosure or mew, followed by examination on the fist, before the "hands-on" physical examination is performed. Clinical signs of cardiovascular disease may vary, but include exercise intolerance, dyspnea, ascites, weakness, neurologic signs, edema of the head and feet, and sudden death. The physical examination should include a complete evaluation of the patient including auscultation of the heart and lungs. Auscultation may reveal arrhythmias, murmurs, and pulmonary congestion, but may be difficult to assess due to the elevated heart rate compared with other species. The veterinarian must be cognizant of the response of the bird to handling, and be prepared to terminate the examination if the patient's condition declines. Dyspnea, ta-chypnea, collapse, syncope, or seizure activity may all warrant termination of the examination. Special attention should be paid to the extremities (especially the tarsus and digits), as swelling is commonly seen in older raptors with cardiovascular disease.

Diagnostic testing may include hematology, biochemistry, radiography, echocardi-ography, endoscopy, electrocardiography, and blood pressure measurement.

Radiographs allow visualization of the heart, aorta, brachiocephalic trunk, and pulmonary vessels. Abnormalities may be seen with the size and shape of the heart, increased radiodensity of large vessels (ie, arteriosclerosis), and enlargement of vessels such as the aorta. Changes in the lungs, liver, and air sacs, secondary to heart disease, may also be noticed, including hepatomegaly, increased radiodensity of the lungs, pleural effusion, and ascites. Measurement of heart length is difficult to assess due to the superimposition of the apex of the heart over the liver. Recommendations for psittacines have been made, which involve measurement of the heart silhouette on ventrodorsal radiographs at its maximum width compared with the width of the thorax

Table 2
Neoplasia reports in birds of prey

Tumor	Number of Cases in the Literature	Species	Average Age	Age Range	References
Fibrosarcoma	17	Multiple species	6.9 y	6 mo to 12 y	94
Myxofibroma	1	Cape griffon vulture	17 y	17 y	94
Fibroma	1	European kestrel	Unknown	Unknown	94
Histiocytic carcinoma	2	Great horned owl	<1 y and one adult	<1 y and one adult	94
Lipoma	4	Multiple species	13 y	9–16 y	94
Osteosarcoma	2	Hybrid falcon, Eurasian buzzard	Unknown	Unknown to adult	94
Osteoma/ Chondroma	4	Multiple species	13 y	6–15 y	94
Rhabdomyosarcoma	1	Lappet-faced vulture	19 y	19 y	94
Leiomyoma	2	Golden eagle, peregrine falcon	17 y	17 y	94,95
Mixed cell tumor	1	Seychelles kestrel	30 d	30 d	94
Adenocarcinoma	16	Multiple species	21.4 y	6–26 y	94
Adenoma	1	Multiple species	13.5 y	7–20 y	94
Bile duct carcinoma	3	Multiple species	23 y	13–33 y	94
Cholangiocarcinoma	1	Red-tailed hawk	Unknown	Unknown	96
Cystadenocarcinoma	1	Peregrine falcon	Unknown	Unknown	95
Cholangiocellular carcinoma and renal adenocarcinoma	1	Golden eagle	Unknown	Unknown	97
Carcinoma	5	Multiple species	8 y	18 mo to 2 y	94
Thyroid follicular cystadenoma	1	Crested caracara	7 y	7 y	94
Thyroid cystic fibroadenoma	1	Black-chested Buzzard eagle	>27 y	>27 y	94
Adrenal cortical adenoma	1	Long-crested eagle	20 y	20 y	94
Squamous cell carcinoma	13	Multiple species	8.7 y	4–15 y	94
Epidermoid carcinoma	2	Red-tailed hawk	Unknown	Unknown	94
Papilloma	6	Multiple species	4 y	6 mo to 9 y	94
Hemangioma	1	Peregrine falcon	15 y	15 y	94
Mast cell tumor	3	Multiple owl species	Unknown	Unknown	94
Melanoma	3	Multiple owl species	20 y	10–31 y	94
Astrocytoma	1	Great horned owl			94

(continued on next page)

Table 2 (continued)					
Tumor	Number of Cases in the Literature	Species	Average Age	Age Range	References
Malignant lymphoma	4	Multiple species	12 y	>8–18 y	94
Malignant thymoma	1	Saker falcon	12 y	12 y	94
Lymphoid leukosis	4	Multiple species	2.5 y	3 mo to 3 y	94
Erythoblastosis	1	Gyrfalcon	Unknown	Unknown	94
Lymphosarcoma	3	Multiple species	22 y	22 y	94
Teratoma	1	Eurasian buzzard	10 y	10 y	94
Xanthoma	3	Multiple species	18 y	2 to >40 y	94
Mesothelioma	2	Ferruginous hawk	4.5 y	4–5 y	94

at the same level.[109] In medium-sized psittacines (200–500 g) the width of the cardiac silhouette should be 51% to 61% of the thoracic width. Hanley and colleagues[110] determined that the width of the cardiac silhouette in the Canadian goose was 47% to 57% of the thoracic width, so species variation seems to exist. Radiographic measurements in raptors remain to be evaluated.

Echocardiography allows further evaluation of the heart structure, function, and kinetics. Visualization of the heart is achieved by a ventromedian approach with the patient in a slightly upright position. On occasion feathers must be removed to allow better contact between the probe and the patient. Echocardiography may reveal decreased contractility, increased thickness of heart chambers and vessels, pericardial effusion, and valvular dysfunction. Color flow Doppler greatly improves diagnostic capabilities regarding evaluation of the heart valves. Reference values have been established for psittacines, pigeons, and raptors.[111] Reference values of echocardiograms for raptors are listed in **Table 3**.

Electrocardiography (ECG) may be used for the detection of arrhythmias, conduction disorders, metabolic disorders, and ventricular enlargement. ECG may also be used along with echocardiography to allow measurement at definitive stages of the heart cycle. ECG reference values have been evaluated for multiple Falconiformes and Strigiformes in a study by Burtnick and Degernes.[112] Reference values of ECG for raptors are listed in **Table 4**.

Endoscopy is another diagnostic tool used for direct visualization of the heart, great vessels, and cardiovascular associated structures.

Diagnostic evaluation should be used to investigate for primary cardiovascular disease as well as conditions that may result in secondary cardiac disease such as gout and septicemia. Reports of cardiovascular disease in raptors include atherosclerosis, ischemic heart disease, vegetative endocarditis, aortic ruptures, toxemia, myocarditis, pericardial effusion, dilated cardiomyopathy, and neoplasia.

Atherosclerosis has been frequently described in birds of prey. Keymer[113] analyzed over 125 birds of prey and found that 10% of Falconiformes and more than 15% of Strigiformes were afflicted with this form of heart disease. More than 85% of the Falconiformes were older than 10 years and all but one of the Strigiformes was older than 12 years. Finlayson[114] noted that the highest incidence of lipid-containing plaques occurred in Falconiformes, approaching 54% in comparison with 6 other Orders of birds in which incidence was between 20% and 30%. Lesions frequently seen with atherosclerosis primarily affect the brachiocephalic trunk and abdominal aorta, with

Table 3

Electrocardiogram (Lead II) heart rate and duration of ECG intervals under anesthesia with ketamine and xylazine

Common Name	Scientific Name	n	Heart Rate (Beats/min)	P (s)	PR (s)	QRS (s)	QT (s)
Bald eagle	Haliaeetus leucocephalus	20	82 (50–160)	0.041 (0.03–0.06)	0.091 (0.07–0.11)	0.029 (0.02–0.04)	0.135 (0.11–0.165)
Great horned owl	Bubo virginianus	8	111 (100–130)	0.037 (0.03–0.05)	0.086 (0.07–0.1)	0.025 (0.02–0.03)	0.149 (0.125–0.165)
Red-tailed hawk	Buteo jamaicensis	11	122 (80–220)	0.032 (0.02–0.035)	0.071 (0.05–0.09)	0.025 (0.02–0.03)	0.116 (0.08–0.165)
American kestrel	Falco sparverius	8	158 (120–200)	0.03 (0.03–0.035)	0.059 (0.05–0.065)	0.021 (0.015–0.025)	0.099 (0.085–0.12)
Golden eagle	Aquila chrysaetos	2	100 (100)	0.043 (0.04–0.045)	0.09 (0.085–0.095)	0.025 (0.025)	0.142 (0.135–0.15)
Peregrine falcon	Falco peregrinus	2	95 (90–100)	0.035 (0.035)	0.072 (0.07–0.075)	0.025 (0.025)	0.135 (0.125–0.145)
Barred owl	Strix varia	2	120 (100–140)	0.055 (0.05–0.06)	0.105 (0.1–0.11)	0.027 (0.025–0.03)	0.145 (0.14–0.15)
Saw-whet owl	Aegolius acadicus	2	240 (200–280)	0.018 (0.01–0.025)	0.055 (0.05–0.06)	0.02 (0.02)	0.102 (0.085–0.12)
Cooper's hawk	Accipiter cooperii	2	160 (140–180)	0.027 (0.025–0.03)	0.062 (0.055–0.07)	0.025 (0.025)	0.098 (0.095–0.1)
Sharp-shinned hawk	Accipiter striatus	2	220 (200–240)	0.03 (0.03)	0.06 (0.055–0.065)	0.02 (0.02)	0.11 (0.09–0.13)

Data from Burtnick NL, Degernes LA. Electrocardiography on fifty-nine anesthetized convalescing raptors. In: Redig PT, Cooper JE, Remple JD, et al, editors. Raptor biomedicine. Minneapolis: University of Minnesota Press; 1993. p. 111–21.

Table 4
Echocardiographic parameters in raptors

Parameter	Diurnal Raptors Horizontal View	Diurnal Raptors Vertical View
Body mass	720 ± 197	
Left ventricle		
Length systole (mm)	14.7 ± 2.0 male 14.7 ± 4.5 female	17.7 ± 1.2 male 18.2 ± 4.7 female
Length diastole (mm)	16.5 ± 1.8 male 16.3 ± 4.5 female	19.3 ± 1.6 male 20.1 ± 5.2 female
Width systole (mm)	6.1 ± 0.8 male 6.8 ± 1.7 female	6.6 ± 0.9 male 7.7 ± 1.8 female
Width diastole (mm)	7.4 ± 1.0 male 8.3 ± 1.8 female	7.5 ± 1.0 male 8.9 ± 2.1 female
Width fractional shortening (%)	unknown	unknown
Right ventricle		
Length systole (mm)	12.6 ± 1.9 male 13.0 ± 4.6 female	
Length diastole (mm)	13.8 ± 1.8 male 14.2 ± 4.2 female	
Width systole (mm)	2.1 ± 0.5 male 2.2 ± 0.8 female	
Width diastole (mm)	2.5 ± 0.7 male 2.5 ± 1.1 female	
Width fractional shortening (mm)	Unknown	
Interventricular septum		
Thickness systole (mm)	1.8 ± 0.4 male 2.0 ± 0.8 female	
Thickness diastole (mm)	1.9 ± 0.4 male 2.0 ± 0.7 female	
Aorta diameter diastole	2.7 ± 0.4 male 2.9 ± 0.4 female	

Data from Pees M, Krautwald-Jughanns ME. Cardiovascular physiology and disease of pet birds. Vet Clin North Am Exot Anim Prac 2009;12(1):81–97; Boskovic M, Krautwald-Junghanns ME, Failing K, et al. Moglichkeiten und Grenzen echokardiographischer Untersuchungen bei Tag- und Nachtgreifvogeln (Accipitriformes, Falconiformes, Strigiformes). Tierarztl Prax 1995;27:334–41.

similar lesions occurring in the subclavian, carotid, and femoral arteries. Gross necropsy may reveal degenerative changes and decrease in the lumen of the arterial wall by deposits of collagen, cholesterol, or calcium, but in some cases gross post-mortem examination may be unremarkable.[115] Obesity and lack of exercise seem to be predisposing factors.

Infectious causes of heart disease are primarily the result of bacterial infections but may also be caused by fungi and parasites resulting in endocarditis, myocarditis, and pericarditis. Vegetative endocarditis has been reported as a result of bumblefoot caused by frostbite in various species of birds, including raptors.[116] Other infectious causes include salpingitis, nephritis, and hepatitis. Myocarditis may be the result of infections with bacteria, fungi, viruses, and parasites. The protozoan parasite *Sarcocystis* spp has been reported in European sparrowhawks.[72] In addition, histopathological changes consistent with myocarditis were seen in 23 of 38 raptors diagnosed with West Nile virus in a report by Saito and colleagues in 2007.[55]

Metabolic conditions such as gout may also affect cardiac function. Renal and hepatic tissues are frequently affected by visceral gout. Other conditions such as dilated cardiomyopathy and degenerative cardiac disease have been seen in bearded vultures and bald eagles with lead toxicity, respectively.[72]

The limited cases of cardiovascular disease diagnosed antemortem has resulted in few reports of drug use for these disease conditions in raptors. The author has used enalapril on a red-tailed hawk (*Buteo jamaicensis*) and a golden eagle (*Aquila chrysaetos*) at a dose of 0.5 to 1.0 mg/kg every 24 hours by mouth, with no ill effects. Treatment of cardiovascular disease in raptors is an area where much work is still needed.

Organ Failure

Hepatic disease and renal disease are frequently identified disease conditions that affect older raptors, yet there are few reports in the literature.[117] Hepatic and renal disease may be the result of several different origins including infectious, inflammatory, degenerative, metabolic, toxic, and neoplastic conditions. Hepatic diseases commonly include hepatic lipidosis, amyloidosis, mycobacteriosis, viral disease, and toxin accumulation. Renal diseases include amyloidosis, neoplasia, gout, viral disease, and toxin accumulation.

Ocular Disease

Falconers, zoologic institutions, and educational facilities frequently present raptors to veterinarians with ophthalmic disease associated with old age. Most forms of ocular disease in raptors are the result of traumatic injuries, many of which predispose raptors to chronic ocular conditions such as cataracts.[118–121] Early detection, diagnosis, and treatment afford the patient the best chance for a favorable outcome.

History is a vital part of the information required when presented with a bird with an ocular condition. Although many traumatic injuries may occur while hunting or during handling by trainers or staff, it may also occur when the bird is on exhibit or in its mew. In these instances, the exact cause of the injury may not be known and the clinical signs may be the first indication of a problem. Clinical signs may consist of a closed eye, ocular discharge, blepharitis, hyphema, hypopyon, lens luxation, inability to close the eye, and anisocoria. Conditions such as iris discoloration due to chronic inflammation, cataract formation, and blindness may be seen with chronic disease.

Visual examination of the patient should be performed, as stated earlier, before a physical examination is performed. Birds that are not trained to come to the glove may initially need to be examined from a distance. If this occurs, binoculars may be used for initial evaluation of the patient without direct or close contact with the bird. Further, "hands-on" examination of the patient may require the use of an ophthalmoscope, fluorescein dye, a Schirmer tear test (STT), tonometry, slit-lamp biomicroscopy, and indirect ophthalmoscopy. Fluorescein staining is a quick, inexpensive technique that is frequently used for diagnosis of corneal defects from penetrating wounds, toxin exposure, and other corneal injuries.[122] Korbel and Leitenstrofer[123] evaluated the use of a modified STT strip in normal birds of prey and identified reference ranges for Falconiformes and Strigiformes. Reference values for STT in raptors are listed in **Table 5**. Marked decreases in the STT ranges were noted in Strigiformes, likely due to their small or absent orbital lacrimal gland. A wide reference range was reported and recommendations were made to assess birds based on their age, gender, and species differences. Further evaluation of the STT has been evaluated in screech owls and tawny owls.[124,125] Tonometry can also be used for evaluation

Table 5
Lacrimal function of normal eyes measured using a modified Schirmer tear test (STT)

Common Name	Scientific Name	Strip (mm)	No. of Birds	No. of Eyes	STT with Topical Anesthesia (mm/min)	STT without Topical Anesthesia (mm/min)	STT with General Anesthesia (mm/min)
Common kestrel	*Falco tinnunculus*	5	15	30	4.07 ± 2.7	1.96 ± 1.7	2.34 ± 1.5
Falco spp	*Falco spp*	5	12	24	14.44 ± 7.2	4.17 ± 3.1	8.26 ± 4.6
Common buzzard	*Buteo buteo*	5	12	24	11.5 ± 5.4	5.9 ± 3.1	6.81 ± 3.8
Sparrow hawk	*Accipiter nisus*	5	4	8	10.63 ± 4	3.6 ± 1.7	
Strigiformes	Strigiformes	2	6	10	2.7 ± 1.4	1.25 ± 0.6	
Tawny owls	*Strix aluco*	2	Unknown	Unknown	3.2 ± 0.4[a]		
Screech owls	*Megascops asio*	Unknown	21	21	2.0 with a range of 2–6		

[a] It is unknown whether topical or general anesthesia was used in the birds in these studies.

Data from Korbel R, Leitenstorfer P. Clinical estimation of lacrimal function in various bird species using a modified Schirmer tear test. Isr J Vet Med 1996;51: 171–5; Williams DL, Villavincencio CM, Wilson S. Chronic ocular lesions in tawny owls (Strix aluco) injured by road traffic. Vet Rec 2006;159:148–53; Harris MC, Schorling JJ, Herring IP, et al. Ophthalmic examination findings in a colony of Screech owls (Megascops asio). Vet Ophthalmol 2008;11(3):186–92.

of intraocular pressures in raptors with uveitis and glaucoma. Primary and secondary causes of glaucoma have been reported in raptors, with 10 of 13 cases occurring in great horned owls (*Bubo virginianus*).[118,126] Reference ranges have been established for various birds of prey including red-tailed hawks (*Buteo jamaicensis*), Swainson's hawks (*Buteo swainsoni*), golden eagles (*Aquila chrysaetos*), bald eagles (*Haliaeetus leucocephalus*), tawny owls (*Strix aluco*), Eurasian eagle owls (*Bubo bubo*), and great horned owls (*Bubo virginianus*).[127,128] Reference values for intraocular pressures in raptors are listed in **Table 6**. Many clinicians do not frequently perform indirect ophthalmic evaluation; however, it should be strongly considered as it provides visualization of a wide field of view of the retina.

The causes of ophthalmic disease are as numerous for raptors as they are for domestic species. Despite this fact, traumatic events dominate the reports in the literature. Additional reports including degenerative, nutritional, neoplastic, infectious, inflammatory, metabolic, and toxic causes of ocular disease can also be found.[130–133] The most common disease condition seen in geriatric raptors, second only to osteoarthritis, is the development of cataracts. Cataracts can develop in birds due to traumatic, developmental, genetic, toxic, or inflammatory lesions.[134–136] Cataracts may be further classified as traumatic, juvenile, or senile types.[133] Senile cataracts are the second most frequently quoted type of cataract after those resulting from traumatic injuries.[133,137–139] Recommended treatment may be palliative, medical, or surgical. Surgical therapy may be chosen due to the inability to apprehend food, inability to mate, continued self trauma, or other factors that may affect quality of life. Surgical treatment of cataracts has been accomplished by needle aspiration, extracapsular extraction, and ultrasonic phacoemulsification.[129,134,138] Indication for cataract surgery is based on evaluation of the patient for current or preexisting medical conditions, as well as the possibility of acceptable postoperative vision. Assistance by a board certified ophthalmologist is invaluable when formulating a plan before a final determination is made. Although the body of knowledge has increased on ophthalmic conditions in raptors over the last 20 years, additional work is still needed regarding ophthalmic conditions in geriatric raptors.

Neurologic Diseases

Most neurologic disease conditions seen in raptors are related to trauma, toxin ingestion and exposure, or infectious origins, such as West Nile virus. Neoplastic, cardiovascular, metabolic, and idiopathic diseases may also result in clinical signs associated with neurologic disease. In geriatric raptors, neurologic conditions are usually the result of neoplastic, cardiovascular, metabolic, and idiopathic diseases and may result in senility, cerebral ischemic events, seizures, and various other neurologic abnormalities.

Senility is occasionally seen in geriatric raptors under the care of falconers or zoologic institutions. Signs of cognitive dysfunction indicating senility include changes in the sleep/wake cycle, inattention to food, inattention to environment, inability to recognize familiar people or objects, or inability to perform learned behaviors. In other species, neurotransmitters change with age, and this likely also occurs in birds.[140] As animals age, acetylcholinesterase and monoamine oxidase b levels increase as choline aminotransferase and serotonin levels decrease and lipofuscin accumulates in the cytoplasm of the neurons. In addition, the brain becomes chronically hypoxic with age due to arteriocapillary fibrosis and endothelial proliferation. Although these changes have been recognized in other species, to the author's knowledge they have not been evaluated in relation to raptors and other avian species. Ultimately, senility is ruled out by exclusion of other differentials that can be definitively

Table 6
Intraocular pressures in birds of prey

Common Name	Scientific Name	No. of Birds	Method of Tonometry Measurement	Normal/Abnormal	IOP mm Hg (±SD)	References
Barred owl	Strix varia	1	Applanation	Right: anterior lens luxation Left: normal	R: 18 L: 18	129
Great horned owl	Bubo virginianus	1	Applanation	Right: corneal perforation and iris prolapse Left: luxated lens, corneal edema, corneal neovascularization	Unable to acquire L: 34	130
Great horned owl	Bubo virginianus	Unknown	Applanation	Normal	10–14	130
Great horned owl	Bubo virginianus	1	Applanation	Right/Left: blind, episcleral congestion, mydriasis, exposure keratitis, abnormal iridocorneal angles, and curled/atrophied pectinate ligament	R: 42.4 (±5.6) L: 26.4 (±1.8)	126
Great horned owl	Bubo virginianus	3	Applanation	Normal	7.1 (5.2–7.8)	126

Common name	Scientific name	n	Tonometry	Finding	IOP (±SD)	Ref
Tawny owl	Strix aluco	26	Applanation	See below	See below	124
		Unknown	Applanation	Normal	15.6 (±3.4)	124
		Unknown	Applanation	With adnexal lesions	14.2 (±3.6)	124
		Unknown	Applanation	With corneal lesions	18.2 (±5.4)	124
		Unknown	Applanation	Anterior segment inflammatory pathology	7.4 (±4.6)	124
		Unknown	Applanation	Iridio- or cyclodialysis	35.4 (±12.2)	124
		Unknown	Applanation	Lens pathology alone	12.2 (±3.8)	124
		Unknown	Applanation	Posterior segment pathology alone	13.6 (±4.8)	124
Eurasian Eagle owl	Bubo bubo	10	Applanation	Normal	9.35 (±1.81)	128
		10	Rebound	Normal	10.45 (±1.64)	128
Red-tailed hawk	Buteo jamaicensis	10	Applanation	Normal	20.6 (±3.4)	127
Swainson's hawk	Buteo swainsoni	6	Applanation	Normal	20.8 (±2.3)	127
Golden eagle	Aquila chrysaetos	7	Applanation	Normal	21.5 (±3.0)	127
Bald eagle	Haliaeetus leucocephalus	3	Applanation	Normal	20.6 (±2.0)	127
Great horned owl	Bubo virginianus	6	Applanation	Normal	10.8 (±3.6)	127

diagnosed. Record keeping specifically related to the behavioral condition of the bird is the most critical aspect to formulating a differential diagnosis of senility in raptors. Medical therapies are available for humans and canines for the treatment of senility, but these medications have not been evaluated for use in birds.

Seizures, tremors, and other cerebral/cerebellar conditions in geriatric raptors can be caused by neoplastic, metabolic (hepatic encephalopathy), cardiovascular, and idiopathic conditions. As stated earlier, toxic exposure and trauma may result in the majority of neurologic conditions, yet in geriatric birds, age-related changes should result in expansion of the clinicians' differential list. Neoplastic, hepatic, and cardiovascular diseases discussed earlier could each contribute to a patient's neurologic symptoms. Defining whether the neurologic disease is primary or secondary to another condition is crucial to implementing appropriate therapy for the patient. A 26-year-old golden eagle (*Aquila chrysaetos*) with opisthotonos, inappetence, incoordination, and stargazing was evaluated by the author. Only after exclusion of infectious, inflammatory, metabolic, toxic, and traumatic causes, and evaluation by computed tomography of the brain with contrast media, was a definitive diagnosis of a cerebral ischemic event able to be confirmed (**Figs. 10–12**). Other reports of neurologic conditions in raptors have been classified as idiopathic until further work is performed to delineate a definitive diagnosis. Avian vacuolar myelinopathy is a condition with an unknown etiology that has affected bald eagles, a great horned owl, and several species of waterfowl, and has been recognized periodically in North America.[141] Although a neurotoxin is suspected, further investigation is needed. Diagnosis and evaluation of neurologic conditions in geriatric birds is still in its early stages, and extensive work is needed to thoroughly understand the impact of these conditions on the health of raptors under human care.

Reproductive Diseases

Reproductive disease in aged raptors has not received adequate attention in the literature compared with other subjects. Although reproductive diseases are covered in various texts, the effect of age and age-related conditions is poorly understood. The reproductive lifespan of most raptors has not been established, nor have all the factors that influence it been identified. Conditions resulting in secondary effects on mating may also influence fecundity. Osteoarthritis may affect reproductive abilities for both the male and female. The male may be unable to mount the female, and dystocia

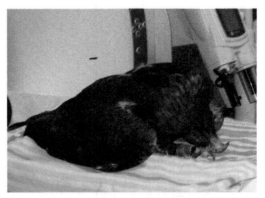

Fig. 10. Golden eagle (*Aquila chrysaetos*) with severe torticollis that was suspected to be due to a cerebral ischemic event. (*Courtesy of* Tim Tristan, DVM.)

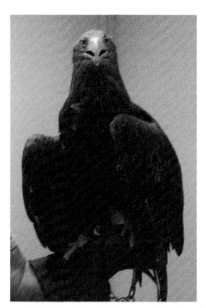

Fig. 11. Full recovery was achieved in the Golden eagle in **Fig. 10** after approximately a month of intense supportive care. (*Courtesy of* Tim Tristan, DVM.)

may become a concern for the female during the egg-laying process. Abnormal plumage near and around the cloaca may also hinder the ability for individuals to copulate. Neoplastic diseases affecting abdominal organs, the reproductive tract, and the cloacal region can also cause problems in reproduction.

Decrease in the reproductive potential of the geriatric male or female can also be primarily associated with the reproductive system. Low sperm counts, decreased sperm volume, decrease sperm motility, and poor sperm morphology are seen in geriatric animals of other species, and need to be taken into consideration with raptors. Decreased receptivity may be observed, and can be a consequence of decreased

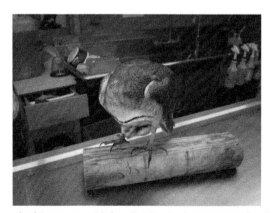

Fig. 12. Many times the history can aid the clinician in determining the diagnosis. This barn owl (*Tyto alba*) with torticollis was due to head trauma from a motor vehicle. (*Courtesy of* Tim Tristan, DVM.)

libido resulting from a drop in hormone production over time for both males and females. Egg production also declines in females partly due to the extensive energy expenditure on the individual. Despite the possible causes of reproductive failure, the effect of age and age-related conditions needs to be more comprehensively examined.

Miscellaneous Conditions

Various other conditions should be considered when caring for geriatric raptors. Age-related changes in other species may result in changes in the immune, integumentary, and respiratory systems. In addition, special attention should be paid to anesthesia and clinical pathologic interpretation.

The immune system and respiratory system each exhibit age-related changes in other species, including humans and canines. A decline in the immune function is seen with many species and can result in increased susceptibility to infectious disease conditions. Alterations in hematology and the biochemical parameters have not been evaluated in geriatric raptors, but may prove critical to a complete understanding of the patient. Age-related decreases in chest wall compliance, pulmonary compliance, and pulmonary elastic fiber properties are seen in dogs with increased age, and this can be appreciated on physical examination and noted by subtle clinical signs of respiratory disease.[142] Similar anatomic and physiologic changes in the respiratory system of geriatric raptors have not been observed to date, and further investigation is warranted. Poor feather quality, including frayed, dull feathers, may be seen in geriatric raptors. Decreased preening due to osteoarthritis or other conditions may affect the health and visual appearance of feathers over time. Other factors including nutrition, infectious agents, and neoplastic disease may also contribute to poor feather quality.

Obesity is frequently seen in elderly raptors in captivity due to decreased activity and overfeeding. Special attention should be made to closely monitor raptor weights to ensure that they remain within their target parameters. Obesity may lead to or exacerbate medical conditions such as osteoarthritis and cardiovascular disease, and eventually may result in decreased life expectancy.

Finally, anesthetic considerations should be accounted for as in other geriatric animals. Complete evaluation of the patient, including physical examination, hematology, biochemistry, and radiographs should be performed to provide baseline data. A thorough workup allows for evaluation of the patient for any underlying or undiagnosed disease conditions that may complicate an anesthetic procedure. Although many clinicians may sedate patients before performing diagnostics, the benefits and risks should be considered before anesthetizing a geriatric bird.

SUMMARY

The limited information available on geriatric raptors emphasizes the extensive effort that is still needed to expand the knowledge and understanding of these specialized patients. Although raptors have been intimately involved with humans for centuries, the medical aspects have lagged behind until recently. Rehabilitation centers have become a major component, allowing a better understanding of medical conditions in raptors, with increased involvement from local veterinarians. Falconers' use of veterinary services has enhanced the care and medical management through a team approach by both disciplines. The improvement in care, husbandry, and medical management at zoologic institutions has and will continue to be a vital component to further understanding of raptors. Ultimately, contributions made by all the groups discussed here will be imperative to the future of geriatric raptor medicine.

ACKNOWLEDGMENTS

The author wishes to acknowledge the Animal Rehabilitation Keep, Downtown Aquarium Houston, and the Texas State Aquarium for their support of conservation efforts in South Texas which has significantly contributed to this publication. In addition, the author expresses sincere appreciation to T.M. Tristan and Amanda Terry for their invaluable assistance in this article.

REFERENCES

1. Redig PT. A decade of progress in raptor medicine. In: Redig PT, Cooper JE, Remple JD, et al, editors. Raptor biomedicine. Minneapolis (MN): University of Minnesota Press; 1993. p. 3–5.
2. Riddle KE, Hoolihan J. A research hospital for falcons: design, operation, and admission summary. In: Redig PT, Cooper JE, Remple JD, et al, editors. Raptor biomedicine. Minneapolis (MN): University of Minnesota Press; 1993. p. 188–93.
3. Rutz C, Whittingham MJ, Newton I. Age-dependent diet choice in an avian top predator. Proc Biol Sci 2006;273:579–86.
4. Bortolotti GR, Smits JE, Bird DM. Iris colour of American kestrels varies with age, sex, and exposure to PCB's. Physiol Biochem Zool 2003;76(1):99–104.
5. Thorup K, Alerstam T, Hake M, et al. Bird orientation: compensation for wind drift in migrating raptors is age dependent. Proc Biol Sci 2003;270(Suppl):S8–11.
6. Ottinger MA, Reed E, Wu J, et al. Establishing appropriate measures for monitoring aging in birds: comparing short and long lived species. Exp Gerontol 2003;38:747–50.
7. Altwegg R, Schuab M, Roulin A. Age-specific fitness components and their temporal variation in the barn owl. Am Nat 2007;169(1):47–61.
8. Martin J, Kitchens WM, Hines JE. Natal location influences movement and survival of a spatially structured population of snail kites. Oecologia 2007;153:291–301.
9. Laaksonen T, Hakkarainen H, Korpimaki E. Lifetime reproduction of a forest-dwelling owl increases with age and area of forests. Proc Biol Sci 2004; 271(Suppl):S461–4.
10. Martell MS, Goggin J, Redig PT. Assessing rehabilitation success of raptors through band returns. In: Lumeij JT, Remple JD, Redig PT, et al, editors. Raptor biomedicine III. Lake Worth (FL): Zoological Education Network; 2000. p. 327–36.
11. Walzer C, Boegel R, Fluch G. Intraabdominal implantation of a multi-sensor telemetry system. In: Lumeij JT, Remple JD, Redig PT, et al, editors. Raptor biomedicine III. Lake Worth (FL): Zoological Education Network; 2000. p. 313–20.
12. Kenward RE, Marcstrom V, Karlbom M. Causes of death in radio-tagged Northern goshawks. In: Redig PT, Cooper JE, Remple JD, et al, editors. Raptor biomedicine. Minneapolis (MN): University of Minnesota Press; 1993. p. 57–61.
13. de Magalhaes JP, Budovsky A, Lehmann G, et al. The human ageing genomic resources: online databases and tools for biogerontologists. Aging Cell 2009; 8(1):65–72.
14. Klimkiewicz MK. Longevity records of North American birds. Version 2008. Laurel (MD): Patuxent Wildlife Research Center, Bird Banding Laboratory; 2008.

15. Heidenreich M. Forensics. In: Birds of prey medicine and management. Oxford (UK): Blackwell, Wissenschafts-Verlag; 1997. p. 231. [Dr Yvonne Oppenheim, Trans.]

16. Dutton CJ, Cooper JE, Allchurch AF. The pathology and diseases of the Mauritius kestrel (Falco punctatus). In: Lumeij JT, Remple JD, Redig PT, et al, editors. Raptor biomedicine III. Lake Worth (FL): Zoological Education Network, Inc; 2000. p. 147–56.

17. Deem SL, Terrell SP, Forrester DJ. A retrospective study of morbidity and mortality of raptors in Florida: 1988–1994. J Zoo Wildl Med 1998;29(2): 160–4.

18. Gottdenker NL, Walsh T, Jimenez-Uzcategui G, et al. Causes of mortality of wild birds submitted to the Charles Darwin Research Station, Santa Cruz, Galapagos, Ecuador from 2002–2004. J Wildl Dis 2008;44(4):1024–31.

19. Muller K, Altenkamp R, Brunnberg L. Morbidity of free-ranging white-tailed sea eagles (Haliaeetus albicilla) in Germany. J Avian Med Surg 2007;21(4):265–74.

20. Wendell MD, Sleeman JM, Kratz G. Retrospective study of morbidity and mortality of raptors admitted to Colorado State University Teaching Hospital during 1995–1998. J Wildl Dis 2002;38(1):101–6.

21. Krone O, Wille F, Kenntner N, et al. Mortality factors, environmental contaminants, and parasites of white-tailed sea eagles from Greenland. Avian Dis 2004;48:417–24.

22. Krone O, Stjernberg T, Kenntner N, et al. Mortality factors, helminth burden, and contaminant residues in white-tailed sea eagles (Haliaeetus albicilla) from Finland. Ambio 2006;35(3):98–104.

23. Harris MC, Sleeman JM. Morbidity and mortality of bald eagles (Haliaeetus leucocephalus) and peregrine falcons (Falco peregrinus) admitted to the wildlife center of Virginia, 1993–2003. J Zoo Wildl Med 2007;38(1):62–6.

24. Kovacs A, Demeter I, Fater I, et al. Current efforts to monitor and conserve the eastern imperial eagle Aquila heliaca in Hungary. Ambio 2008;37(6):457–9.

25. Coone NC, Locke LN, Cromartie E, et al. Causes of bald eagle mortality, 1960–1965. J Wildl Dis 1970;6:72–6.

26. Komnenou AT, Georgopoulou I, Savvas I, et al. A retrospective study of presentation, treatment, and outcome of free-ranging raptors in Greece (1997–2000). J Zoo Wildl Med 2005;36(2):222–8.

27. Punch P. A retrospective study of the success of medical and surgical treatment of wild Australian raptors. Aust Vet J 2001;79(11):747–52.

28. Richards BA, Lickey A, Sleeman JM. Decreasing prevalence and seasonal variation of gunshot trauma in raptors admitted to the wildlife center of Virginia:1993–2002. J Zoo Wildl Med 2005;36(3):485–8.

29. Lumeij JT, Westerhof I. Diagnosis and treatment of poisoning in raptors from the Netherlands: clinical case reports and review of 2,750 postmortem cases, 1975-1988. In: Redig PT, Cooper JE, Remple JD, et al, editors. Raptor biomedicine. Minneapolis (MN): University of Minnesota Press; 1993. p. 233–8.

30. Nakamaru M, Iwasa Y, Nakanishi J. Extinction risk to bird populations caused by DDT exposure. Chemosphere 2003;53:377–87.

31. Garcia-Fernandez AJ, Motas-Guzman M, Maria-Mojica NP, et al. Environmental exposure and distribution of lead in four species of raptors in Southeastern Spain. Arch Environ Contam Toxicol 1997;33:76–82.

32. Miller MJR, Restani M, Harmata AP, et al. A comparison of blood lead levels in bald eagles from two regions on the great plains of North America. J Wildl Dis 1998;34(4):704–14.

33. Saito K, Kurosawa N, Shimura R. Lead poisoning in endangered sea-eagles (*Haliaeetus albicilla, Haliaeetus pelagicus*) in Eastern Hokkaido through ingestion of shot sika deer (*Cervus nipon*). In: Lumeij JT, Remple JD, Redig PT, et al, editors. Raptor Biomedicine III. Lake Worth (FL): Zoological Education Network; 2000. p. 163–8.

34. Zaccaroni A, Amorena M, Naso B, et al. Cadmium, chromium and lead contamination of *Athene noctua*, the little owl, of Bologna and Parma, Italy. Chemosphere 2003;52:1251–8.

35. Meteyer CU, Rideout BA, Gildert M, et al. Pathology and proposed pathophysiology of Diclofenac poisoning in free-living and experimentally exposed Oriental white-backed vultures (*Gyps bengalensis*). J Wildl Dis 2005;41(4): 707–16.

36. Oaks JL, Gilbert M, Virani MZ, et al. Diclofenac residues as the cause of vulture population decline in Pakistan. Nature 2004;427:630–3.

37. White DH, Hayes LE, Bush PB. Case histories of wild birds killed intentionally with famphur in Georgia and West Virginia. J Wildl Dis 1989;25(2): 184–8.

38. Dietz R, Riget FF, Boertmann D, et al. Time trends of mercury in feathers of West Greenland birds of prey during 1851-2003. Environ Sci Technol 2006;40: 5911–6.

39. Elliot JE, Langelier KM, Mineau P, et al. Poisoning of bald eagles and red-tailed hawks by carbofuran and fensulfothion in the Fraser Delta of British Columbia, Canada. J Wildl Dis 1996;32(3):486–91.

40. Kenntner N, Tataruch F, Krone O. Heavy metals in soft tissue of white-tailed sea eagles found dead or moribund in Germany and Austria from 1993-2000. Environ Toxicol Chem 2001;20(8):1831–7.

41. Kenntner N, Krone O, Altenkamp R, et al. Environmental contaminants in liver and kidney of free-ranging Northern goshawks (*Accipiter gentilis*) from three regions of Germany. Arch Environ Contam Toxicol 2003;45:128–35.

42. Kenntner N, Krone O, Oehme G, et al. Organochlorine contaminants in body tissue of free-ranging white-tailed eagles from Northern regions of Germany. Environ Toxicol Chem 2003;22(7):1457–64.

43. Knopper LD, Mineau P, Walker LA, et al. Bone density and breaking strength in UK raptors exposed to second generation anticoagulant rodenticides. Bull Environ Contam Toxicol 2007;78:249–51.

44. Zuberogoitia I, Martinez JA, Ireata A, et al. Short-term effects of the prestige oil spill on the peregrine falcon (*Falco peregrinus*). Mar Pollut Bull 2006;52: 1176–81.

45. Hakkarainen H, Korpimaki E, Laaksonen T, et al. Survival of male Tengmalm's owls increases with cover of old forest in their territory. Oecologia 2008;155:479–86.

46. Haas D. Clinical signs and treatment of large birds injured by electrocution. In: Redig PT, Cooper JE, Remple JD, et al, editors. Raptor biomedicine. Minneapolis (MN): University of Minnesota Press; 1993. p. 180–3.

47. Altwegg R, Roulin A, Kestenholz M. Demographic effects of extreme winter weather in the barn owl. Oecologia 2006;149:44–51.

48. Sarasola JH, Negro JJ, Salvador V, et al. Hailstorms as a cause of mass mortality of Swainson's hawks in their wintering grounds. J Wildl Dis 2005;41(3):643–6.

49. Wiens JD, Noon BR, Reynolds RT. Post-fledging survival of northern goshawks: the importance of prey abundance, weather, and dispersal. Ecol Appl 2006; 16(1):406–18.

50. Heckel JO, Sisson DC, Quist CF. Apparent fatal snakebite in three hawks. J Wildl Dis 1994;30(4):616–9.
51. Ziman M, Colagross-Schouten A, Griffey S, et al. *Haemoproteus* spp. and *Leukocytozoon* spp. in a captive raptor population. J Wildl Dis 2004;40(1):137–40.
52. Green CH, Gartrell BD, Charleston WAG. Serratospiculosis in a New Zealand falcon (*Falco novaeseelandiae*). N Z Vet J 2006;54(4):198–201.
53. Szabo KA, Mense MG, Lipscomb TP, et al. Fatal toxoplasmosis in a bald eagle (*Haliaeetus leucocephalus*). J Parasitol 2004;90(4):907–8.
54. Gancz AY, Barker IK, Lindsay R, et al. West Nile virus outbreak in North American owls, Ontario, 2002. Emerg Infect Dis 2004;10(12):2135–42.
55. Saito EK, Sileo L, Green DE, et al. Raptor mortality due to West Nile virus in the United States, 2002. J Wildl Dis 2007;43(2):206–13.
56. Nemeth NM, Beckett S, Edwards E, et al. Avian mortality surveillance for West Nile virus in Colorado. Am J Trop Med Hyg 2007;76(3):431–7.
57. Wunschmann A, Shivers J, Bender J, et al. Pathologic findings in red-tailed hawks (*Buteo jamaicensis*) and Cooper's hawks (*Accipiter cooperi*) naturally infected with West Nile virus. Avian Dis 2004;48:570–80.
58. Pinkerton ME, Wellehan JFX, Johnson AJ, et al. Columid herpesvirus-1 in two Cooper's hawks (*Accipiter cooperii*) with fatal inclusion body disease. J Wildl Dis 2008;44(3):622–8.
59. Tomaszewski EK, Phalen DN. Falcon adenovirus in an American kestrel (*Falco sparverius*). J Avian Med Surg 2007;21(2):135–9.
60. Kenward R. The causes of death in trained raptors. In: Cooper JE, Greenwood AG, editors. Recent advances in the study of raptor diseases. Keighley. West Yorkshire (UK): Chiron Publications Ltd; 1981. p. 27–9.
61. Kenward R. Mortality and fate of trained birds of prey. J Wildl Manag 1974;38: 751–6.
62. Rothschild BM, Panza R. Osteoarthritis is for the birds. Clin Rheumatol 2006;25: 645–7.
63. Cooper JE. Miscellaneous and emerging diseases. In: Birds of prey: health and disease. 3rd edition. Oxford (UK): Blackwell Science Ltd; 2002. p. 185–216.
64. Samour J. Raptors. In: Harrison GJ, Lightfoot TL, editors, Clinical avian medicine. Palm Beach (FL): Spix publishing Inc; 2006;2: p. 915–56.
65. Graham JE, Kollias-Baker C, Craigmill AL, et al. Pharmacokinetics of ketoprofen in Japanese quail (*Coturnix japonica*). J Vet Pharmacol Ther 2005;28: 399–402.
66. Baert K, De Backer P. Comparative pharmacokinetics of three non-steroidal anti-inflammatory drugs in five bird species. Comp Biochem Pysiol C Toxicol Pharmicol 2003;134:25–33.
67. Wilson GH, Hernandez-Divers SJ, Budsberg SC, et al. Pharmacokinetics and use of meloxicam in psittacines birds. In: Proc Assoc Avian Vet Conf. New Orleans (LA); August 17–19, 2004. p. 7–9.
68. Machin KL, Teller LA, Lair S, et al. Pharmacodynamics of flunixin and ketoprofen in mallard ducks (*Anas platyrhynchus*). J Zoo Wildl Med 2001;32: 222–9.
69. McGeown D, Danbury TC, Waterman-Pearson AE, et al. Effect of carprofen on lameness in broiler chickens. Vet Rec 1999;144:668–71.
70. Danbury TC, Weeks CA, Chambers JP, et al. Self-selection of the analgesic drug carprofen by lame broiler chickens. Vet Rec 2000;146:307–11.

71. Baert K, De Backer P. Disposition of sodium salicylate, flunixin, and meloxicam after intravenous administration in ostriches (*Struthio camelus*). J Avian Med Surg 2002;16:123–8.
72. Jones R. Raptors: systemic and non-infectious diseases. In: Chitty J, editor. BSAVA manual of raptors, pigeons, and waterfowl. Ames (IA): Iowa State University Press; 2008. p. 284–98.
73. Dahlhausen R, Aldred S, Colaizzi E. Resolution of proventicular dilatation disease by cyclooxygenase 2 inhibition. In: Proc Assoc Avian Vet. Monterey (CA); August 26–30, 2002. p. 9–12.
74. Paul-Murphy J, Hess JC, Fiakowski JP. Pharmacokinetic properties of a single intramuscular dose of buprenorphine in African grey parrots (*Psittacus erithacus erithacus*). J Avian Med Surg 2004;18:224–8.
75. Hoppes S, Flammer K, Hoersch K, et al. Disposition and analgesic effects of fentanyl in white cockatoos (*Cacatua alba*). J Avian Med Surg 2003;17: 124–30.
76. Schneider C. Effects of morphine-like drugs in chicks. Nature 1961;191:607–8.
77. Hughes RA. Strain-dependent morphine-induced analgesic and hyperalgesic effects on thermal nociception in domestic fowl (*Gallus gallus*). Behav Neurosci 1990;104:619–24.
78. Hughes RA. Codeine analgesia and morphine hyperalgesia effects on thermal nociception in domestic fowl. Pharmacol Biochem Behav 1990;35:567–70.
79. Fan SG, Shutt AJ, Vogt M. The importance of 5-hydroxytryptamine turnover for the analgesic effect of morphine in the chicken. Neuroscience 1981;6: 2223–7.
80. Gentle MJ, Hocking PM, Bernard R, et al. Evaluation of intraarticular opioid analgesia for the relief of articular pain in the domestic fowl. Pharmacol Biochem Behav 1999;63:339–43.
81. Paul-Murphy J, Brunson DB, Miletic V. Analgesic effects of butorphanol and buprenorphine in conscious African grey parrots (*Psittacus erithacus erithacus*). Am J Vet Res 1999;60:1218–21.
82. Curro TG. Evaluation of the isoflurane sparing effects of butorphanol and flunixin in psittaciformes. In: Proc Assoc Avian Vet. Monterey (CA); August 26–30, 2002. p. 17–19.
83. Curro TG, Brunson DB, Paul Murphy J. Determination of the ED50 of isoflurane-sparing effects of butorphanol in cockatoos (*Cacatua* spp.). Vet Surg 1994;23: 429–33.
84. Riggs SM, Hawkins MG, Craigmill AL, et al. Pharmacokinetics of butorphanol tartrate in red-tailed hawks (*Buteo jamaicensis*) and great horned owls (*Bubo virginianus*). Am J Vet Res 2008;69(5):596–603.
85. Heatley JJ. Anaesthesia and analgesia. In: Chitty J, editor. BSAVA manual of raptors, pigeons, and waterfowl. Ames (IA): Iowa State University Press; 2008. p. 97–113.
86. Kukanich B, Papich MG. Pharmacokinetics of tramadol and O-esmethyltramadol in dogs. J Vet Pharmacol Ther 2004;27:239–46.
87. Souza MJ, Jones MP, Cox SA. Pharmacokinetics of tramadol in bald eagles (*Haliaeetus leucocephalus*). In: Proc Assoc Avian Vet. Providence (RI); August 6–9, 2007. p. 7–8.
88. Stevenson R. Cosequin for old Amazon. Exotic Dvm 1999;1(1):34.
89. Robertson S. Osteoarthritis in cats: what we now know about recognition and treatment. Vet Med 2008;103(11):611–6.

90. Tully TN. Avian dermatology. In: Proc West Vet Conf. Las Vegas (NV); February 11–14, 2002.

91. Lightfoot TL. Feather "Plucking". Atlantic Coast Veterinary Conference. Atlantic City (NJ); October 9–11, 2001.

92. Doneley B. The use of gabapentin to treat presumed neuralgia in a little corella (*Cacatua sanguinea*). In: Proc Assoc Avian Vet Aust Comm. Melbourne (Australia); 2007.

93. Siperstein LJ. Use of Neutontin (Gabapentin) to treat leg twitching/foot mutilation in a Senegal parrot. In: Proc Assoc Avian Vet. Providence (RI); August 6–9, 2007. p. 81–2.

94. Forbes NA, Cooper JE, Higgins RJ. Neoplasms in birds of prey. In: Lumeij JT, Remple JD, Redig PT, et al, editors. Raptor biomedicine III. Lake Worth (FL): Zoological Education Network; 2000. p. 127–46.

95. Montijano MG, Lopez IL, Eiguren AA, et al. Cystadenocarcinoma and leiomyoma in a peregrine falcon (*Falco peregrinus brookei*). Vet Rec 2008;162:859–61.

96. Hartup BK, Steinberg H, Forrest LJ. Cholangiocarcinoma in a red-tailed hawk (*Buteo jamaicensis*). J Zoo Wildl Med 1996;27:539–43.

97. Mikaelian I, Patenaude R, Girard C, et al. Metastatic cholangiocellular carcinoma and renal adenocarcinoma in a golden eagle (*Aquila chrysaetos*). Avian Pathol 1998;27:321–5.

98. Doolen M. Adriamycin chemotherapy in a blue-front amazon with osteosarcoma. In: Proc Assoc Avian Vet. Reno (NV); September 28–30, 1994. p. 89–91.

99. Ramsey EC, Bos JH, McFadden C. Use of cisplatin and orthovoltage radiotherapy in treatment of a fibrosarcoma in a macaw. J Assoc Avian Vet 1993; 7(2):87–90.

100. Kollias GV, Homer B, Thompson JP. Cutaneous psuedolymphoma in a juvenile blue and gold macaw (*Ara ararauna*). J Zoo Wildl Med 1992;23(2):235–40.

101. France M, Gilson S. Chemotherapy treatment of lymphosarcoma in a Moluccan cockatoo. In: Proc Annu Conf Assoc Avian Vet. Nashville (TN); August 31 to September 4, 1993. p. 15–19.

102. Zantop DW. Treatment of bile dust carcinoma in birds with carboplatin. Exotic Dvm 2000;2(3):76–8.

103. Speer BL, Eckermann-Ross C. Diagnosis and clinical management of pancreatic duct adenocarcinoma in a green-winged macaw (Ara chloroptera). In: Proc Eur Conf Avian Med Surg. Munich (Germany); 2001. p. 225.

104. Filippich LJ, Bucher AM, Charles BG, et al. Intravenous cisplatin administration in sulfur-crested cockatoos (*Cacatua galerita*): clinical and pathological observations. J Avian Med Surg 2001;15(1):23–30.

105. Lamberski N, Theon A. Concurrent irradiation and intratumoral chemotherapy with cisplatin for treatment of a fibrosarcoma in a blue and gold macaw (*Ara ararauna*). J Avian Med Surg 2002;16(3):234–8.

106. Freeman KP, Hahn KA, Adams WH, et al. Radiation therapy for hemangiosarcoma in a budgerigar. J Avian Med Surg 1999;13(1):40–4.

107. Rosenthal K, Duda L, Ivey ES, et al. A report of photodynamic therapy for squamous cell carcinoma in a cockatiel. In: Proceedings of the 22nd Annual AAV Conference. Orlando (FL); August 22–24, 2001. p. 175–6.

108. Heatley JJ, Bellah J, Brawner J, et al. Radiation therapy of squamous cell carcinoma in a golden eagle. In: Proc Assoc Avian Vet. Providence (RI); August 6–9, 2007. p. 327–8.

109. Straub J, Pees M, Krautwald-Junghanns ME. Measurement of the cardiac silhouette in psittacines. J Am Vet Med Assoc 2002;221:76–9.

110. Hanley CS, Helen GM, Torrey S, et al. Establishing cardiac measurement standards in three avian species. J Avian Med Surg 1997;11:15–9.
111. Pees M, Krautwald-Jughanns ME. Cardiovascular physiology and disease of pet birds. Vet Clin North Am Exot Anim Pract 2009;12(1):81–97.
112. Burtnick NL, Degernes LA. Electrocardiography on fifty-nine anesthetized convalescing raptors. In: Redig PT, Cooper JE, Remple JD, et al, editors. Raptor biomedicine. Minneapolis (MN): University of Minnesota Press; 1993. p. 111–21.
113. Keymer IF. Disease of birds of prey. Vet Rec 1972;90:579–94.
114. Finlayson R. Vascular disease in captive animals. Symposium of the Zoological Society of London, vol. 11. London (UK): Academic Press; 1964. p. 99–106.
115. Shrubsole-Cockwill A, Wojnarowicz C, Parker D. Atherosclerosis and ischemic cardiomyopathy in a captive, adult red-tailed hawk (Buteo jamaicensis). Avian Dis 2008;52:537–9.
116. Wallach JD, Flieg GM. Frostbite and its sequelae in captive exotic birds. J Am Vet Med Assoc 1969;155(7):1035–8.
117. Lumeij JT. Pathophysiology, diagnosis and treatment of renal disorders in birds of prey. In: Lumeij JT, Remple JD, Redig PT, et al, editors. Raptor biomedicine III. Lake Worth (FL): Zoological Education Network; 2000. p. 169–78.
118. Murphy CJ, Kern TJ, McKeever K, et al. Ocular lesions in free-living raptors. J Am Vet Med Assoc 1982;181(11):1302–4.
119. Murphy CJ, Kern TJ, Riis RC. Intraocular trauma in a red-tailed hawk. J Am Vet Med Assoc 1982;181(11):1390–1.
120. Korbel RT. Disorders of the posterior eye segment in raptors—examination procedures and findings. In: Lumeij JT, Remple JD, Redig PT, et al, editors. Raptor biomedicine III. Lake Worth (FL): Zoological Education Network; 2000. p. 179–94.
121. Scope A, Fery H. Diseases and mortality causes in captive and free-ranging bearded vulture (Gypaetus barbatus). In: Lumeij JT, Remple JD, Redig PT, et al, editors. Raptor biomedicine III. Lake Worth (FL): Zoological Education Network; 2000. p. 327–36.
122. Murphy CJ, Kern TJ, MacCoy DM. Bilateral keratopathy in a Barred owl. J Am Vet Med Assoc 1981;179(11):1271–3.
123. Korbel R, Leitenstorfer P. Clinical estimation of lacrimal function in various bird species using a modified Schirmer tear test. Isr J Vet Med 1996;51: 171–5.
124. Williams DL, Villavincencio CM, Wilson S. Chronic ocular lesions in tawny owls (Strix aluco) injured by road traffic. Vet Rec 2006;159:148–53.
125. Harris MC, Schorling JJ, Herring IP, et al. Ophthalmic examination findings in a colony of Screech owls (Megascops asio). Vet Ophthalmol 2008;11(3):186–92.
126. Rayment LJ, Williams D. Glaucoma in a captive-bred great horned owl (Bubo virginianus virginianus). Vet Rec 1997;140:481–3.
127. Stiles J, Buyukmihci NC, Farver TB. Tonometry of normal eyes in raptors. Am J Vet Res 1994;55(4):477–9.
128. Jeong MB, Kim YJ, Yi NY, et al. Comparison of the rebound tonometer (TonoVet) with the applanation tonometer (TonoPen XL) in normal Eurasian eagle owls (Bubo bubo). Vet Ophthalmol 2007;10(6):376–9.
129. Brooks DE, Murphy CJ, Quesenberry KE, et al. Surgical correction of a luxated cataractous lens in a barred owl. J Am Vet Med Assoc 1983;183(11): 1298–9.

130. MacLaren NE, Krohne SG, Porter RE, et al. *Corynebacterium* endophthalmitis, glaucoma, and scleral ossicle osteomyelitis in a great horned owl (*Bubo virginianus*). J Zoo Wildl Med 1995;26(3):453–9.

131. Murphy CJ, Kern TJ, Loew E, et al. Retinal dysplasia in a hybrid falcon. J Am Vet Med Assoc 1985;187(11):1208–9.

132. Buyukmihci NC, Murphy CJ, Schulz T. Developmental ocular disease of raptors. J Wildl Dis 1988;24(2):207–13.

133. Murphy CJ. Raptor ophthalmology. Comp Contin Educ 1987;9(3):241–60.

134. Carter RT, Murphy CJ, Stuhr CM, et al. Bilateral phacoemulsification and intraocular lens implantation in a great horned owl. J Am Vet Med Assoc 2007; 230(4):559–61.

135. Canton DD, Murphy CJ, Buyukmihci NC, et al. Pupilloplasty in a great horned owl with papillary occlusion and cataracts. J Am Vet Med Assoc 1992;201(7): 1087–90.

136. Brooks DE. Avian cataracts. Semin Avian Exotic Pet Med 1997;6(3):131–7.

137. Keymer IF. Cataracts in birds. Avian Pathol 1977;6:335–41.

138. Kern TJ, Murphy CJ, Riis RC. Lens extraction by phacoemulsification in two raptors. J Am Vet Med Assoc 1984;185(11):1403–6.

139. Moore CP, Pickett JP, Beehler B. Extracapsular extraction of senile cataract in an Andean Condor. J Am Vet Med Assoc 1985;187(11):1211–3.

140. Goldston RT. Introduction and overview of geriatrics. In: Goldston RT, Hoskins JD, editors. Geriatrics and gerontology of the dog and cat. Philadelphia: W.B. Saunders; 1995. p. 1–9.

141. Fischer JR, Lewis-Weis LA, Tate CM, et al. Avian vacuolar myelinopathy outbreaks at a southeastern reservoir. J Wildl Dis 2006;42(3):501–10.

142. Taboada J. The respiratory system. In: Goldston RT, Hoskins JD, editors. Geriatrics and gerontology of the dog and cat. Philadelphia: W.B. Saunders; 1995. p. 63–88.

Diseases of Geriatric Guinea Pigs and Chinchillas

Jeffrey R. Jenkins, DVM, DABVP (Avian)

KEYWORDS

- Guinea pig • Chinchilla • Geriatric • Scurvy
- Pododermatitis • Malocclusion

In the United States over the last 10 years, interest has been increasing in small mammal pets, including guinea pigs and chinchillas. This trend has resulted in improved diet and husbandry, which in turn has led to increased longevity of many of these pets. The problems and diseases of the older guinea pig and chinchilla differ to some extent from that of the young newly obtained animal, although diet and husbandry still play important roles.

The guinea pig (*Cavia porcellus*), or cavy, is a species of rodent belonging to the family Caviidae and the genus *Cavia*. They are believed to have been domesticated by natives of the Andean region of South America over 5000 years ago. The animals are thought to be descendants of a closely related species, *Cavia aperea*, *Cavia fulgida*, or *Cavia tschudii*, and therefore do not exist naturally in the wild.[1] The guinea pig still plays an important role as a food source and in folk medicine and religious ceremonies in this part of the world.[2]

The chinchilla (*Chinchilla laniger*) was introduced to Spaniards in 1524 and named after the Chinchas Indians, a once great nation that had been absorbed into the Inca, who named the animals *Chinchillas*, meaning *little Chinchas*. The demand for chinchilla pelts that followed drove the chinchilla close to extinction and, in 1910, the hunting or exportation of chinchillas was outlawed.[3] According to an apocryphal legend, all of the chinchillas in North America originated from 11 animals—8 males and 3 females—of mixed species (*C laniger* and *Chinchilla brevicaudata*) collected from several different locations and brought to the United States by Mathias F. Chapman in 1923. True or not, the resultant animal is a marvel of physiology. Not only is it the longest living rodent of its size, but it is also remarkably healthy, with only a handful of health problems, most related to poor diet or husbandry.

The aged guinea pig suffers from a long list of diseases and problems. Most important is hypovitaminosis C. Several other problems are directly or indirectly influenced

Avian & Exotic Animal Hospital Inc, 2317 Hotel Circle South, Suite C, San Diego, CA 92108-3310, USA
E-mail address: drexotic@aol.com

Vet Clin Exot Anim 13 (2010) 85–93
doi:10.1016/j.cvex.2009.12.004
1094-9194/10/$ – see front matter © 2010 Published by Elsevier Inc.

by low vitamin C levels, including dental disease and pododermatitis. Dental disease in guinea pigs may be associated with skull size and jaw length as this problem is more prevalent in short-faced animals. Chinchillas have very few old-age disease problems. Both species suffer from renal disease in their last years and many die of complications of kidney failure.

PROBLEMS OF DIET AND HUSBANDRY

Inappropriate diet and husbandry is a major cause of problems for the older guinea pig. Hypovitaminosis C (scurvy) is the most common cause of death in the author's practice and likely contributes to many other health problems of older guinea pigs, including malocclusion, arthritis, and tissue mineralization. Soiled or inappropriate bedding or housing surfaces contribute to pododermatitis, urinary tract infections, and vaginal and scrotal plugs.

Hypovitaminosis C (Scurvy)

Guinea pigs lack the hepatic enzyme 1-gulonolactone oxidase, which is essential for the conversion of glucose to ascorbic acid, a sugar acid with antioxidant properties. The name *ascorbic acid* is derived from *a*, meaning *no*, and *scorbutus*, the medical term for scurvy. Vitamin C is involved in many biochemical processes in the body, including the synthesis of collagen and intracellular ground substance. If vitamin C is not supplemented in the diet, or if the animal is anorexic, scorbutic lesions will rapidly develop.

Clinical signs associated with scurvy vary widely, depending on the level of vitamin C in the diet. Diets containing no vitamin C lead to a more rapidly progressing form of the disease with acutely painful joints and teeth that result in generalized immobility and prevent the consumption of food. The common presentation seen with marginal levels of vitamin C is a chronic form of disease. Signs include frequent vocalizations, weakness, decreased mobility, anorexia, diarrhea, flaky to ulcerative skin lesions, stiffness, petechia of the mucous membranes, subcutaneous hemorrhages, and death due to starvation or secondary infection. Other nonspecific but suspicious signs may include rough hair coat, delayed wound healing, worsening or recurrence of unapparent dermatophyte or scabies infections, changes in patterns of teeth grinding, inactivity, stillbirths, urine scald, and recurrent or chronic disease, including pneumonia and urinary tract infections.[4]

A tentative diagnosis is made based on symptoms and dietary history, while a more definitive diagnosis can be made by analysis of diet, gross and microscopic pathology, and serum ascorbate levels.

Scurvy can be prevented in the guinea pig by supplementing the diet with vitamin C. The daily requirement of ascorbic acid is 15 to 30 mg per guinea pig per day. Pregnant females should receive 30 to 45 mg/d. The author prefers vitamin C supplements added to the drinking water (the author recommends Liquid C [Twin Lab, American Fork, Utah, UT, USA]). Because of instability of vitamin C in the presence of light and chlorine, a solution at a concentration of 200 to 400 mg/L drinking water should be mixed fresh daily. Supplemental feeding of a cup of cabbage, kale, a whole green pepper, or similar foods may be sufficient. However, results are unreliable.

Commercial guinea pig diets are formulated with supplementary vitamin C. The typical feed pellets contain 800 mg/kg at the time of milling. Such factors as dampness, heat, and light can reduce the vitamin C content during storage. Even pellet diets stored under optimal conditions lose their potency within 90 days of milling.[5]

Commercial pet diets may have a shorter storage life — 30 to 60 days after milling — and are not a dependable source of vitamin C.

Pododermatitis

Pododermatitis includes a range of lesions of the weight-supporting palmar or plantar surfaces of the feet. Trauma to the foot, caused by wire floors or rough bedding, results in inflammation, atrophy of epithelium, infection, fibrous proliferation, loss of vascularization, necrosis, and then granuloma formation, tendonitis, and osteomyelitis of one or more footpads. Untreated, lesions infiltrate vital structures, resulting in lameness, loss of function, and eventually the death of the animal. *Staphylococcus aureus* is frequently isolated from lesions, entering the skin through cracks from abrasions or exposure to moisture. Predisposing factors include obesity, rough or wire flooring, poor sanitation, and other trauma. In the author's opinion chronic cases may progress to lymphadenopathy, arthritis, tendonitis, and amyloid accumulation in kidneys, liver, adrenal glands, spleen, and pancreatic islets.

Diagnosis of pododermatitis is based on clinical signs. Prognosis is based on a five-level classification taken from that for birds of prey, reported by Remple[6]:

Level I: Lesions involve skin only, no infection or inflammation of underlying tissues, and may be divided into two subclasses: hyperemic and hyperkeratotic.

Level II: Lesions involve skin and the subcutaneous tissues but no gross tissue swelling. Again this level is divided into those with obvious trauma and those with ischemic necrosis of the weight-bearing surface.

Level III: The feet are swollen and painful without obvious involvement of deep tissues. This level is divided into three subclasses based on inflammation: serous, fibrotic, or caseous.

Level IV: Infection extends into deep or vital tissues, but the patient retains normal pedal use of the foot. This is evidence of chronicity. This level may be subdivided once again into two subclasses: fibrotic and caseous lesions.

Level V: Normal pedal function is lost. Infection, inflammation, and tissue destruction has extended into tendon, bone, and joints, resulting in crippling deformities, loss of function, and a grave prognosis.

Medical Treatment

Only the mildest cases of bumblefoot should be treated with medical treatment alone. These would include level I and level II lesions. Healing is slow and lesions may recur or progress. Change bedding to absorbent underpads or sheet liners. Culture lesions and administer appropriate antibiotics. Treat lesions topically with silver sulfadiazine cream (SSD) (Silvadine Cream 1% [Monarch Pharmaceuticals, Inc, Bristol, TN, USA]). Systemic antibiotics, such as azithromycin at 40 mg/kg every 24 hours (Zithromax [Pfizer Inc, New York, NY, USA]) should be administered and modified based on culture results. Treatment must be continued until lesions have healed, which may take weeks to months. Bandaging or a combination of bandages and protective "shoe" dressings may be required for more severe lesions to heal.

Surgery is indicated for level III or greater lesions. Surgery decreases convalescence time in many cases and may improve prognosis. If a single limb is involved with an advanced (level IV or V) lesion, amputation is indicated.

Before surgery, take radiographs to assess bone involvement and prognosis. Osteomyelitis/arthritis adversely affects prognosis for recovery. Treat medically for 2 to 4 weeks before surgery to reduce inflammation and vascularity and to improve long-term prognosis. Buprenorphine and meloxicam are given before induction of anesthesia and continued for several days postoperatively. Self-adherent bandaging tape (Vetrap Bandaging Tape [3M, St Paul, MN, USA]), cut into a 1-in strip, is wrapped above the elbow/hock as a tourniquet. Wrap just tight enough to take the wrinkles out of the tape to control bleeding without damaging the circulation or nerves of the leg. Clean the feet gently but thoroughly to remove any soil, shedding skin, and debris, and remove any scab.

Using an electrosurgical, radiosurgical, or laser surgical device, make an incision around the lesion. Remove all necrotic tissue and the fibrous capsule of the lesion, and trim skin to full thickness with bleeding edges. Take care to avoid vessels and nerves. Curette to remove any necrotic tissue and irrigate to remove any debris. Close incision in a manner that best retains normal foot architecture and prevents skin from constricting the foot. Use small, 5-0 to 7-0, monofilament absorbable or nylon suture. Place simple interrupted and vertical mattress sutures alternately, beginning and ending with simple interrupted.

Following surgery, bandage the foot using a shoe dressing. A hole is made in the shoe to prevent pressure on the closure and enable visualization of the incision. A variety of materials may be used to create the shoe, including polymethyl methacrylate resin (Jet Denture Repair Acrylic [Lang Dental Manufacturing Co Inc, Wheeling, IL, USA]), thermoplastic casting tape, padded aluminum splint (SAM splint [Jorgensen Laboratories, Loveland, CO, USA]), cotton cast padding, or rubber foam. The shoe should cover the palmar/plantar foot and extend up the posterior lower leg at an angle comfortable for standing.

Postsurgical management includes daily assessment of bandaging and appropriate antibiotics for 2 to 3 weeks. At 2 to 3 weeks, remove shoe bandages and simple continuous sutures. Apply a light-weight bandage over SSD cream (human Band-Aid bandages work well). At 3 to 4 weeks, remove mattress sutures and continue bandaging and SSD for an additional 7 days.

Prognosis is based on the level of the lesion. Level I carries a favorable prognosis with aggressive treatment. Level II and III carry a good prognosis, and level IV lesions have a guarded to poor prognosis. Level IV lesions have a poor to grave prognosis for saving the limb. Consider amputation in vivacious animals. Manage others with analgesics, such as meloxicam at 0.3 mg/kg every 12 hours (Metacam [Boehringer Ingelheim, St Joseph, MO, USA]), and long-term antibiotics therapy.

Spurs

"Spurs" are growths of calluses that form on the lateral side of the carpal foot pad. Some breeds and heavy-bodied animals are more prone to developing spurs, and wire or hard-surface cage flooring appears to contribute as well. These growths may get long, exceeding 0.5 cm, and may contribute to cracks in the carpal pad that develop into pododermatitis. Carefully trim these spurs and file smooth with a fine grit emery board or nail buffer. Reduction of body weight, correction of caging/bedding, and regular application of lotion or softening agent to carpal pads reduce the likelihood of recurrence.

Cheek Tooth Overgrowth and Malocclusion

Chinchillas and guinea pigs have both open-rooted incisors and cheek teeth.[7,8] They are classified as full elodonts.[9] All of the teeth grow continuously, which makes these rodents more susceptible to malocclusion, which in turn leads to conditions that affect the animal's general health.

Guinea pigs and chinchillas grow and wear several inches of teeth annually. If for any reason they are unable to wear their teeth at the rate that they grow, problems develop.

While diet plays a role in tooth wear, the primary force affecting tooth wear is occlusion and bruxing (grinding of the teeth). It is the opposing tooth or teeth that wear rodent teeth. If the excursion of the jaw is limited, or if bruxing is painful, then tooth wear is limited or nonexistent and tooth spurs form or teeth lengthen. If lateral movement of the mandible is not sufficient to cover the opposing cheek teeth, the mandibular cheek teeth wear to form lingual spurs, whereas the maxillary teeth form buccal spurs.[8] Elongated maxillary spurs cause lacerations of the cheeks, while elongated mandibular spurs can form an arch, trapping the tongue. With guinea pigs, this problem of elongated mandibular spurs is often complicated by a collapsing of mandibular cheek teeth associated with loss of periodontal ligaments secondary to scurvy.

Nutrition, genetics, and trauma may play roles in the development of dental pathology. Scurvy, as mentioned above, likely plays a major role in the problem in guinea pigs. Dental pain, resulting from damage to periodontal ligaments and loose teeth, results in the animal not chewing vigorously or long enough to adequately keep up with the rate of growth. The teeth are not worn adequately and overgrow results in tongue entrapment and a mouth that is unable to close. Trauma to teeth caused by external forces, such as falling, or that caused by chewing hard objects, may cause uneven wear and result in overgrowth or formation of spurs.

Clinical signs of cheek-tooth malocclusion include oral pain, anorexia, weight loss, salivation ("slobbers"), "open mouth," incisor malocclusion and overgrowth, facial abscesses, exophthalmos, and ocular discharge. Diagnosis is based on signs, oral examination, and radiographs. Clinicians should obtain well-positioned rostrocaudal and lateral views to examine the occlusal plane and temporomandibular joints, along with right and left oblique views to evaluate for problems of elongated roots, periodontal disease, osteomyelitis, or abscessation. The presence of any of these problems denotes a poorer prognosis.

Treatment should address underlying disease, prevent oral pain, and reestablish normal occlusion. Anesthesia is required for oral examination and the trimming of cheek teeth. Cheek teeth have less enamel than do incisors and may be carefully trimmed with a sharp pair of rongeurs or with a tapered bit on a narrow dental drill. Care must be taken not to damage soft tissues while trimming teeth. For many of these patients, the trimming of their teeth is only a means of treating the symptoms of the underlying problem. For an overwhelming number of these patients, a cure is not possible.

Prognosis in these cases varies with the underlying cause, severity, and duration of the problem. Mild cases of cheek-tooth spurs addressed early have a good prognosis.

Chinchillas are not affected by scurvy, but they do have problems with tooth wear as a complication secondary to having short, brachiocephalic faces. Short-faced chinchillas often have crowding of cheek teeth and resulting impaction, oral pain, elongation of tooth roots, and movement of cheek-tooth location, leading to impaired tooth wear and the formation of dental spurs. Some chinchillas presented with signs of cheek-tooth problems will be found on oral examination to have normal-appearing teeth with well-worn occlusal tables. Radiographs of these animals show dental impaction. Many of these patients will stop salivating and begin eating with the administration of analgesia. "Rocking" these patients' cheek teeth with an elevator may help alleviate oral pain. Others appear to "grow out" of the problem over a 2- to 6-week period.

Vaginitis and Scrotal Plugs

Wood chips may adhere to the vulva and vestibule, or to the prepuce of guinea pigs, causing a foreign body reaction. Male guinea pigs may accumulate a plug of sebaceous material, feces, and bedding in the skin fold overlying the interscrotal septum. Treat both conditions by washing the affected area with detergent and water, carefully removing debris. If infected, take cultures and treat the area topically with SSD and administer systemic antibiotics. Problem animals should be placed on a different surface, such as underpads, towels, or waterproof bed pads.

PROBLEMS NOT ASSOCIATED WITH DIET OR HUSBANDRY

Guinea pigs and chinchillas suffer a variety of problems related to metabolism, infection, or just old age. Some of these problems, such as diabetes mellitus and ovarian cysts, may occur in young animals. However, they are more consistently associated with age.

Diabetes Mellitus

Spontaneous diabetes mellitus was first reported in Abyssinian guinea pigs in 1973.[10,11] The disease resembles juvenile diabetes in humans. Studies suggest an infectious cause. About half of a group of females developed diabetes mellitus 6 weeks to 3 months after they were introduced into a colony as breeders.[12] In a group of six guinea pigs, three developed diabetes mellitus over a 12-month period (Jeffrey R. Jenkins, DVM, personal observation, 2001). Other studies showed plaques in embryonated eggs inoculated with urine of affected guinea pigs and found viral particles resembling type C retrovirus.[12]

In a research environment, signs of guinea pig diabetes mellitus most often are seen by 6 months of age. In practice, signs are more commonly seen in mid- to late life. Most often, affected animals show signs of polydipsia, polyuria, and weight loss. Diagnosis is based on abnormal blood glucose levels, glucose tolerance tests, and glucosuria. Affected guinea pigs commonly have urine glucose of greater than 250 mg/dL. Cases treated by the author often have sustained blood glucose levels over 1000 mg/dL. Diabetic guinea pigs do not develop ketoacidosis. Some guinea pigs may have a regression of signs associated with regeneration of beta cells over a period of months to years (unpublished observation).

According to reports, guinea pig diabetes has been successfully treated with insulin. Doses have been based both on glucose levels and normalizing signs of polyuria and polydipsia. The author has used longer acting forms or combinations of long- and short-acting forms. Care must be taken and treatment customized to the patient and the owner's schedule. The author has had a single highly successful case of a guinea pig treated with glipizide at 2 to 5 mg/kg every 12 hours. This animal's owner was highly motivated and followed glucose levels, adjusting the dose as needed. Treatment was continued for over 2 years, at which time glucose levels had returned to normal.

Diabetes mellitus has been reported in chinchillas only three times, and has been linked to obesity. In two cases, animals showed blood glucose levels elevated to at least four times the upper limit of the reference range, as well as severe glycosuria and ketonuria. The animals were treated with insulin and, after initial improvement, both animals died. In the third case, diabetes was at first suspected because of the high blood glucose level and glycosuria, although typical findings, such as ketonuria, polyuria, polydipsia, obesity, and cataracts, were not present. In addition, the serum fructosamine level did not appear to be elevated. The suspected diabetes mellitus in the third case was at first treated with glipizide, 2.5 mg per animal every 12 hours, to stimulate endogenous insulin release (T.M. Donelly, Veterinary Information Network discussion board, May 4, 2009, personal observation).

A single blood glucose concentration measurement is not sufficient for a diagnosis of diabetes mellitus in rodents. Several measurements are required because stress, pain, hyperthermia, and shock can all cause hyperglycemia.

Ovarian Cysts/Rete Cystadenoma

Serous cysts (cystadenoma), originating from cells of the ovarian rete, form in the ovaries of guinea pigs. These cysts have been shown to form in guinea pigs as young as 10 days old and increase in size with age.[13] They are present in all guinea pigs over 1 year of age.[14] In aged guinea pigs, these cysts may be very large. The author has removed cysts measuring greater than 5 cm. Large cysts may affect the function of other organs and the ability to eat a sufficient volume of food.

Clinically, ovarian cysts are associated with signs of depression, anorexia, alopecia, reduced reproductive performance, cystic endometrial hyperplasia, mucometra, and endometritis. As female guinea pigs age, a significant percentage develop a bilateral alopecia. Although no one has proved that the cysts cause the alopecia, the alopecia resolves if an ovariohysterectomy is performed.

Metastatic Calcification

Often asymptomatic, metastatic calcification occurs primarily in mature male guinea pigs.[15] Clinical signs may include weight loss, muscle and joint stiffness, renal failure, or sudden death. Lesions include calcium deposits in the lungs, major organs, the gastrointestinal tract, joints, and skeletal muscles. Organ mineralization is said to be related to diets high in calcium and phosphorus and low in magnesium and potassium. Metastatic calcification is uncommon in guinea pigs fed a diet of hay and green leafy vegetables.

Renal Failure

Perhaps the most common manner in which guinea pigs and chinchillas "die of old age" is renal failure. These patients are typically presented for weight loss, polydipsia/polyuria, or urine scald. Initially laboratory findings include isosthenuria and proteinuria. Only as the disease progresses are blood chemistry values suggestive of renal failure, including elevated blood urea nitrogen and creatinine. In advanced cases, there may be a significant proteinuria, glucosuria, and hematuria. With time, these patients can lose a large portion of their muscle mass and eventually die of primary renal disease or secondary complications.

Trichofolliculoma

Trichofolliculomas are the most common skin tumors of guinea pigs. Two major reviews showed that 45% and 38% of all skin tumors were trichofolliculomas.[16,17] They are benign tumors of the hair follicle epithelium that present as slow-growing cystic masses varying in diameter from 0.5 to 7 cm. They are located predominantly on the back, sides, and lateral thighs. Males are reported to be affected twice as frequently as females. Trichofolliculomas may be found on young guinea pigs, but are most common on animals 3 years and older. Ulcerating tumors and ruptured cysts discharge caseous material. Epidermoid cysts arising from hair follicles are often associated with these tumors, or may arise independently. Treatment is surgical excision.

Other Neoplasms

Guinea pigs and chinchillas have a lower than average frequency of neoplasms.[18]

Guinea pigs

The most common reproductive tumor of guinea pigs is the uterine leiomyoma, which is usually associated with cystic rete ovarii.[19,20] The most common ovarian tumor of guinea pigs is the unilateral teratoma, usually seen in sows over 3 years of age. These benign tumors rarely metastasize. Both male and female guinea pigs can present with mammary tumors, most commonly benign fibroadenomas, but approximately 30% are locally invasive adenocarcinomas that rarely metastasize.[21] The most common respiratory tumor of guinea pigs is bronchogenic papillary adenoma, reported as 30% to 35% of all neoplasms in guinea pigs over 3 years of age. Also, bronchogenic and alveologenic adenocarcinomas have been documented.[22]

Chinchillas

Only a handful of tumors have been reported in chinchillas in the literature. These tumors include lymphoma, uterine leiomyosarcoma, osteosarcoma, and adenocarcinoma of the lung. The author has seen a number of other tumors over the past 25 years. However, there are no notable trends.[23]

REFERENCES

1. Weir BJ. Notes on the origin of the domestic guinea-pig. In: Rowlands IW, Weir BJ, editors. Symposia of the Zoological Society of London, Number 34. The biology of hystricomorph rodents. London (UK): Academic Press; 1974. p. 437–46. Nowak, Ronald M. (1999). p. 437–46.
2. Morales E. The guinea pig: healing, food, and ritual in the andes. Tucson (AZ): University of Arizona Press; 1995.
3. Mitchell MA, Tully TN. Manual of exotic pet practice. Saint Louis (MO): Elsevier Health Sciences; 2008.
4. Clarke GL, Allen AM, Small JD, et al. Subclinical scurvy in the guinea pig. Vet Pathol 1980;17:40–4.
5. Cheeke PR. Rabbit feeding and nutrition; chapter 19—nutrition of guinea pigs. Orlando (FL): Academic Press, Inc; 1987. p. 349.
6. Remple JD. Raptor bumblefoot: a new treatment technique. In: Redig PT, Cooper JE, Remple JD, et al, editors. Raptor biomedicine. Minneapolis (MN): University of Minnesota Press; 1993. p. 154–60.
7. Wiggs RB, Lobprise H. Dental disease in rodents. J Vet Dent 1990;7(Sept):6–7.
8. Legendre LFJ. Malocclusions in guinea pigs, chinchillas and rabbits. Can Vet J 2002;43(5):385–90.
9. Kertesz P. Veterinary dentistry and oral surgery. London: Wolfe Pbl; 1993. p. 36.
10. Balk MW, Lang CM, White WJ, et al. Exocrine pancreatic dysfunction in guinea pigs with diabetes mellitus. Lab Invest 1975;32:28–32.
11. Lang M, Munger BL. Diabetes mellitus in the guinea pig. Diabetes 1976;25: 434–43.
12. Lee KJ, Lang CM, Munger BL. Isolation of virus-like particles from the urine of guinea pigs (Cavia porcellus) with spontaneous diabetes mellitus. Vet Pathol 1978;15(5):663–6.
13. Nielsen TD, Holt S, Ruelokke ML, et al. Ovarian cysts in guinea pigs: influence of age and reproductive status on prevalence and size. J Small Anim Pract 2003; 44(6):257–60.
14. Quattropani SL. Serous cysts of the aging guinea pig ovary I. Light microscopy and origin. Anat Rec 2005;188(3):351–9.

15. O'Rourke DP. Disease problems of guinea pigs. In: Quesenberry KE, Carpenter JW, editors. Ferrets, rabbits, and rodents clinical medicine and surgery. 2nd edition. Philadelphia: Saunders; 2004. p. 245–54.

16. Frank H, Frese K. Trichofollikulome beim Meerschweinchen [Trichofolliculomas in guinea pigs]. Tierarztliche Umschau 1988;43:242–8 [in German].

17. Ediger RD, Kovatch RM. Spontaneous tumours in the Dunkin-Hartley guinea pig. J Natl Cancer Inst 1976;56:293–4.

18. Greenacre CB. Spontaneous tumors of small mammals. Vet Clin North Am Exot Anim Pract 2004;7(3):627–51.

19. Harkness JE, Wagner JE. Specific diseases and conditions. In: Harkness JE, Wagner JE, editors. The biology and medicine of rabbits and rodents. 4th edition. Philadelphia: Williams and Wilkins; 1995. p. 171–322.

20. Field KJ, Griffith JW, Lang CM. Spontaneous reproductive tract leiomyomas in aged guinea pigs. J Comp Pathol 1989;101:287–94.

21. Collins BR. Common diseases and medical management of rodents and lagomorphs. In: Jacobson ER, Kollias GV, editors. Exotic animals. New York: Churchill Livingstone; 1988. p. 261–316.

22. Harkness JE, Wagner JE. Specific diseases and conditions. In: Harkness JE, Wagner JE, editors. The biology and medicine of rabbits and rodents. 4th edition. Philadelphia: Williams and Wilkins; 1995. p. 171–322.

23. Simova-Curd S, Nitzl D, Pospischil A, et al. Lumbar osteosarcoma in a chinchilla (Chinchilla laniger). J Small Anim Pract 2008;49(9):483–5.

The Ancient Rat

Vicky L. Haines, DVM, DACLAM[a,b,*]

KEYWORDS

• Geriatric • Rat • Disease • Husbandry

The past decade has seen an increase in the number of rodents being kept as pets and subsequently in the number of rodent owners seeking veterinary services. The American Veterinary Medical Association (AVMA) reported more than 3 million pet rodents in their 2007 US Pet Ownership & Demographics Sourcebook, nearly double the number reported in the 2001 statistics.[1,2] These new miniature "companion animals" have the advantage of being inexpensive to maintain and easily and humanely housed with a minimum of space. The common rat (*Rattus norvegicus*) has become increasingly popular, particularly as novel varieties/genetic mutations have been introduced to the pet market. The average laboratory or domestic pet rat has a life expectancy of approximately 2.5 to 3 years, although 4 years and longer have been reported.[3] Rats are intelligent, trainable, and are responsive to, and even seek out attention from, their caregivers. This behavior emulates that of more traditional companion animals and supports the formation of the human animal bond. Rat owners will seek out quality veterinary medical care to improve and extend the life of their pet. As with traditional companion animals, such as the dog and cat, the aged rat is susceptible to various geriatric diseases, many of which are analogous to geriatric canine and feline maladies. The type and frequency of disease may vary with the strain, stock, or variety of rat.[3]

This article describes disease processes, diagnostics, therapeutics, and husbandry management in the aging rat. The diseases described are not intended to be all inclusive but to represent some of the more common findings. Most of the information on diseases, disease pathology, procedures, and pharmaceutical recommendations and dosages are derived from laboratory animal medicine. Many of the procedural and pharmaceutical recommendations are based on empirical dose ranges extrapolated from other species, trial and error in the laboratory setting, and anecdotal reports. Rat/rodent pet owners should be advised of this and be made aware of potential risks involved in treatment of their pets, particularly in a compromised geriatric animal. References for rodent therapeutics may be found in *The Veterinary Clinics of North*

[a] Texas A&M Institute for Preclinical Studies, Texas A&M University, Mail Stop 44748, College Station, TX 77843-44748, USA
[b] Department of Veterinary Small Animal Clinical Sciences, College of Veterinary Medicine, Texas A&M University, TX, USA
* Corresponding author. Texas A&M Institute for Preclinical Studies, Texas A&M University, Mail Stop 44748, College Station, TX 77843–44748.
E-mail address: vhaines@tamu.edu

Vet Clin Exot Anim 13 (2010) 95–105
doi:10.1016/j.cvex.2009.09.001
1094-9194/10/$ – see front matter © 2010 Elsevier Inc. All rights reserved.

America, Exotic Animal Practice,[36] the *ACLAM Formulary for Laboratory Animals*, 3rd edition,[9] and the *Exotic Animal Formulary*, 3rd edition.[10]

Basic physiology and anatomy, symptoms of disease, and methods for physical examination of the rat have been covered by others.[3–5] In the geriatric rat, particular attention should be paid to gait, stiffness and coordination, "lumps and bumps," respiratory effort, evidence of ascites, and fecal or urinary soiling. Porphyrin pigment, a red discoloration, may be seen around the eyes and nares in a stressed or compromised rat of any age. **Table 1** includes a synopsis of normal rat physiologic data.

RENAL DISEASE

Chronic progressive nephrosis/nephropathy (PGN, CPN) is one of the more common causes of death in aged rats and the incidence has been reported as high as 75% in some strains (Sprague Dawley).[6] The disease occurs more frequently in males and is generally of greater severity than the disease in females. Gross lesions of CPN may be found as early as 6 months of age in some strains of rats but housing and diet may play a significant role in incidence. Early gross lesions of the disease demonstrate classic cortical surface pitting. As the disease progresses, interstitial fibrosis, segmental glomerulosclerosis, dilation of cortical and medullary tubules with eosinophilic proteinaceous casts and secondary hyperparathyroidism with dystrophic mineralization in the kidney, gastrointestinal tract, lungs, and large arteries may be found. Hypertension, ascites, and polyarteritis nodosa have been associated with late-stage disease.[3,6] Rats may have severe disease, seem to compensate well, then suddenly decompensate and die. Weight loss, lethargy, and proteinuria (>20 mg/dL) may be the only overt symptoms.[7,8] The astute owner may note polydypsia or polyuria. (Normal urine production in a healthy rat in a 24-hour period is approximately 5.5 mL/100 g body weight; water consumption per 24-hour period is 8–12 mL/100 g body weight)[3,9] Blood chemistry evaluation may reveal increased blood urea nitrogen and creatinine levels, decreased serum albumin/globulin ratio, and hypercholesterolemia. Glomerular filtration rate (GFR) may be decreased by 25% in very aged rats (30 months or greater).[8,9] Differential diagnoses should include chronic bacterial pyelonephritis, congenital hydronephrosis, ischemic injury, and toxic nephrosis.[6]

Diagnostics

Rats and mice typically urinate when handled. Free catch urine samples may be obtained in this way during examination. Alternatively, the bladder is generally easily palpated in the nonobese rat and a bladder tap may be performed using a 25-gauge 0.5-inch needle. Preferably, the fur on the abdomen should be shaved (a battery-operated

Table 1
Data compiled from Laboratory animal medicine, 2nd edition[3] and the Exotic animal formulary, 3rd edition[9]

Heart rate	300–500 beats/min
Blood volume	6.0–6.4 mL/100 g body weight
Respiratory rate	85 respirations/min
Body temperature	37.5°C
Food consumption/24 h	5–6 g/100 g body weight
Water consumption/24 h	8–12 ml/100 g body weight
Basal metabolism rate (400 g rat)	35 kcal/24 h

moustache clipper with a 1-inch blade works well and creates minimal noise) and the skin disinfected before needle tap. An assistant can gently restrain the rat on its back using one hand to restrain the head and forelimbs and the other to extend the rear limbs. The rat's head should be pointed slightly downward to displace the intestines cranially. The bladder may then be digitally isolated with a thumb and forefinger for sampling. Fractious animals should be sedated. The ventral prostate is large and bilobed in the male rat. It lies over the base and neck of the bladder and may completely cover a small bladder. Care should be taken not to hit the prostate and a bladder tap should not be attempted if the bladder is not easily isolated. **Table 2** details reference ranges for normal rat urine.

Blood work may also be performed, although traditional experimental sites for blood collection in the rat, such as orbital bleeds or laceration of tail vessels, may not be aesthetically pleasing in the clinical situation. The lateral caudal tail vein can be easily accessed for obtaining blood samples and administration of fluids and therapeutics. Commercial laboratory rat restrainers, guillotine cones, or towels wrapped around the rat may be used to assist manual restraint during collection. Care should be taken not to restrict the thorax or obstruct the nares and mouth. Isoflurane anesthesia via chamber/facemask may be necessary or advantageous: chamber sedation (3%–4% isoflurane in 100% oxygen) followed by 1.5% to 2% isoflurane in 100% oxygen via facemask. Facemasks may be fashioned from syringe cases. A latex glove finger or dental damn material may be used as a diaphragm over the end. Small cable ties may be used to secure the diaphragm to the cone. Sevoflurane may be preferred to isoflurane, and has worked well in compromised rats because of its rapid induction and emergence from anesthesia. (Sharmon Hoppes, DVM, Texas A&M, College Station, Texas, August 2009, personal communication.) Additional information on anesthesia of rodents may be found in *The Veterinary Clinics of North America, Exotic Animal Practice,*[40] *Anesthesia and Analgesia in Laboratory Animals,*[38] and *Laboratory Animal Anesthesia.*[39] The tail vein may be accessed using a 1-inch 21- or 23-gauge catheter or needle and the blood sample may be obtained by insertion of a capillary tube into the hub of the needle or catheter. Alternatively a few drops of blood may be dripped into a microtainer. The dorsal tarsal vein may also be accessed in the rat. A 27-gauge needle is recommended; 500–1000 μL can be safely taken from the average adult (250 g or more) rat and divided between ethylenediaminetetraacetic acid (EDTA) and serum microtainer tubes. Generally, a single maximum blood draw of 5.5 mL/kg of rat is safe, with a 2-week recovery period before repeating.[10]

Prevention

Laboratory rat strains such as the Sprague Dawley and Fischer 344, known to have increased incidence of CPN, have decreased incidence and severity when on 25%

Table 2 Data created from Laboratory animal medicine, 2nd edition[3] and the Exotic animal formulary, 3rd edition[9]	
Urine volume/24 h	5.5 mL/100 g body weight
Urine pH	7.3–8.5
Urine specific gravity	1.022–1.070
Protein	<20 mg/dL; <30 mg/dL
Urine osmolarity	1659 mOsm/kg of H_2O
Urine Na$^+$:K$^+$ excretion/24 h	1.63 mEq; 0.83 mEq/100 g body weight

to 30% reduction in caloric intake, relative to ad libitum feeding.[11] It is thought that overfeeding results in prolonged increased renal blood flow and GFR.[12] Although some inbred laboratory strains of rats have been fed commercial rodent diets (protein concentration of 22%–25%) ad libitum, without development of significant renal disease, prevention of overfeeding in pet rats may help to delay the onset and decrease the incidence of CPN.[8]

Treatment

As with the aged dog or cat, treatment is palliative. Lowering the protein content in the diet and supplemental fluids for "stressed" rats may ameliorate the situation temporarily (0.9% saline or 50:50 saline/lactated Ringer solution; dosed at 50–100 mL/kg/24 h maintenance dose warmed to body temperature[9]). Recommended dosage volume for fluids is 25 mL/kg maximum per subcutaneous administration; 10–25 mL/kg maximum per intraperitoneal administration using a 25- and 23-gauge needle, respectively.[10] Reducing dietary protein levels lower than 20% to 10% to 14% may also be advantageous.[8] Angiotensin-converting enzyme (ACE) inhibitors have been suggested for associated hypertension.[13]

Nephrocalcinosis (deposition of calcium phosphate in the kidneys) is also seen in aged rats. It is more common female rats and incidence varies with the strain/stock. High levels of dietary calcium or phosphorus, low calcium/phosphorus ratios, or low magnesium may contribute to the disease incidence. Mineral deposition is generally observed histologically at the corticomedullary junction.[3] Clinically advanced cases may demonstrate renal dysfunction, including albuminuria.[6]

GENITOURINARY DISEASE

Urinary calculi of the renal pelvis and urinary bladder has been reported and may be associated with hematuria, cystitis, hydronephrosis, and obstruction. Calculi have been composed of ammonium magnesium phosphate, mixed carbonate and oxalate, and mixed carbonate and phosphate with magnesium and calcium.[14] Water restriction may be associated with formation of calculi.[6] Calculi may occasionally be seen at the tip of the penis and be gently milked out. A small 23- to 25-gauge flexible intravenous catheter may be used as a urinary catheter to back flush obstructive calculi into the bladder to relieve obstruction. Extremely gentle manipulation and plenty of lubricant are required, and a few drops of lidocaine may be mixed in the flushing solution. In the male, the penis should be manually extruded, and after the catheter is placed into the tip the penis should be extended distally to allow advancement over the pubic area. Surgical intervention (cystotomy) may be successfully performed. Supplemental subcutaneous fluids, antibiotics, heat source, and analgesia should be provided. Choice of antibiotics, analgesics, and fluids from referenced sources should be made with consideration of the extent of organ compromise involved. Calculi should not be confused with vesical proteinaceous plugs, secretions from the accessory sex glands of the rat that may also be seen at the tip of the penis or refluxed back into the bladder. In aged rats, these secretions may become hardened and cause irritation and obstruction.

Male Genital Track

Preputial gland adenitis is common in rats older than 12 months.[15] Gland ducts may be distended with inspissated secretion and necrotic debris, and abscesses may also occur. Draining abcesses can be flushed with antibiotic/steroid salves or mild antibacterial solutions. Systemic antibiotics may be administered in more severe cases. Prostatic hyperplasia and prostatic adenocarcinomas have been seen.[8] Surgical debulking of the prostate, which has multiple lobes in the rat, including tissue ventral, dorsal, lateral to the urethra, and tissue ventral to the seminal vesicle, is a difficult surgery requiring intensive postoperative supportive care. Small tumors located solely in the ventral prostate or seminal vesicle have the best chance for resection but owners should be cautioned that they will most likely return. Prostatic tumors may lead to obstruction of urine flow from the bladder. Testicular atrophy, interstitial (Leydig) cell tumors, dystrophic calcification in degenerating tubules, and polyarteritis nodosa of testicular arteries are also seen in the aged male rat.[8]

Female Genital Track

After 9 months of age, litter size decreases, and the pregnancy rate declines after 12 months of age. Fetal wastage may be as high as 65% by 11 months of age.[3] Hydrometra, pyometra, and cystic endometrial hyperplasia have been reported.[16,17] Surgical intervention, (ovariohysterectomy)may be performed if the rat is otherwise stable.[18] Perioperative analgesics, antibiotics, supplemental heat, and fluid therapy are essential.

MYOCARDIAL DISEASE

Cardiomyopathy has been found to be a major cause of death in aged male rats (>1 year), although there may be no obvious signs of cardiac insufficiency. Twenty-five percent or more of rats of some strains may be affected. Moderate-to-marked ventricular hypertrophy and pale streaks may be visible on gross necropsy. Necrosis of myocardial fibers and infiltration of mononuclear cells are seen histopathologically. The papillary muscles and interventricular septum are most commonly affected.[3,6] Dietary restriction (25%–30% of total caloric intake ad libitum) has been shown to reduce the incidence of this disease in rats.[19] Therapy is supportive, although experimentally, ACE and zinc metalloproteinase inhibitors have been used successfully, to prevent left ventricular remodeling and systolic dysfunction by inhibiting matrix metalloproteinase (MMP-2) activation.[20,21]

DERMATOLOGIC

Thinning and loss of hair, yellowing of the hair in albino strains because of sebum accumulation in the skin and scaley discolored tails may be seen.[22] Yellow material accumulating on the tail and adjacent to the ear may darken with time, possibly from oxidation or bacterial action. Male rats also accumulate brown-pigmented "scales" on the skin over the dorsum, tail, and perineum. These scales overlay normal color skin and can be removed. It has been suggested that these scales may be oxidized lipid or amino acids. Gonadectomy/castration can be "curative."[3] Orchiectomy of rodents has been described elsewhere but of particular note in the rat is that the inguinal canal must be closed after removal of the testes.[18]

ALVEOLAR HISTIOCYTOSIS

Alveolar histiocytosis is a common incidental necropsy finding in the lungs of aged rats and should not be mistaken for viral pneumonia of rats. Grossly it appears as white-to-tan foci approximately 1 mm in diameter, on the pleural surface. Microscopically subpleural accumulation of foamy macrophages may be seen. The cause is unknown.[3]

POLYARTERITIS NODOSA AND ATHEROSCLEROSIS

Polyarteritis nodosa is a chronic progressive disease of aging rats, occurring in medium-size arteries of the mesentery, pancreas, pancreaticoduodenal artery and testis. It is a spontaneous disease seen more frequently in males of certain strains (Sprague Dawley and spontaneously hypertensive rats) or in rats with late-stage nephropathy.[6] Atherosclerosis of the aorta, carotids, and coronary arteries may develop in older rats, and has been associated with intensive breeding (siring or whelping 5 or 6 litters in a 9- to 12-month period). Atherosclerosis may not be linked with myocardial degeneration in the rat, but significant coronary artery disease has been linked with acute subendocardial infarction in the rat.[23]

LIVER PATHOLOGY

Bile ductular proliferation and extramedullary hematopoiesis have been seen in older rats.[6]

RETINAL DEGENERATION

Although not specifically an aging change, retinal degeneration is seen in albino rats subjected to light intensities of 130 lux or greater, intensities that are generally harmless to rats with pigmented uveal tracts. Because this is a progressive disease, caused by gradual reduction of the photoreceptor cell nuclei in the outer nuclear layer of the central retina, apparent disturbances in sight or subsequent cataract formation from this may be noted in older rats.[6] Owners with albino rats should be aware of light sensitivity in their pets.

DEGENERATIVE OSTEOARTHRITIS

Articular cartilage erosion of the sternum and femur is seen in aged rats. Osteoarthritis of the tibiotarsal joints and medial femoral condyles is also sporadically seen.[5,6] Decubital ulcers of the plantar surfaces of the hind feet may be seen in aged obese rats housed on wire. Severe cases may lead to chronic periostitis and osteitis. Chronic spondylitis is also seen in geriatric rats. Nonsteroidal antiinflammatories such as meloxicam, carprofen, or flunixin meglumine may offer relief from arthritis. Recommended dosages are varied and therapy may require tailoring the dose to the individual case.[9,10,24,25]

CENTRAL NERVOUS SYSTEM DEGENERATIVE CHANGES

Posterior weakness, disturbances in motor function, including tail dragging, or paresis in the aged rat may indicate radicuoloneuropathy, a degenerative disease of the spinal roots accompanied by atrophy of skeletal muscle in the lumbar region and hind limbs.[24] Incidence in older rats (>24 months) may be as high as 75% to 90%. Demyelination and vacuolation are seen in the lumbosacral roots, most notably in the ventral spinal regions.[6,25] Although no nutritional component has been defined, some advocate supplementation with B complex. B vitamins have been shown to attenuate inflammatory and neuropathic pain effectively in experimental animals.[26–28] Oral and parental forms of B vitamins have been used.

Focal Wallerian degeneration of the spinal cord and segmental demyelination of peripheral nerves, particularly the sciatic nerves, has also been noted. Degeneration of neurons in the brain and spinal cord have also been noted in aged rats.[29]

SKELETAL MUSCLE

Muscles of the hind quarters, especially the gastrocnemius and adductor, may become atrophic and flabby in the geriatric rat. Rats affected by muscular degeneration may have difficulty in using their rear limbs, develop posterior paresis, paralysis, loss of tail control, urinary incontinence, or atony. Weight loss may also be noted. Histologically, individual muscle fibers are decreased in diameter and there is a prominence of sarcolemmal nuclei secondary to hypertrophy and hyperplasia.[8] It has been suggested that the skeletal muscle lesions are caused by neurogenic atrophy secondary to nerve root and spinal cord lesions (radiculoneuropathy), although skeletal muscle lesions are delayed by caloric restriction and radiculoneuropathy is not.[30,31]

Aged rats suffering from arthritis, neuro, or muscular disease need to be monitored closely to ensure that they are able to access food and water sources with ease. Traction mats or additional bedding material on the bottom of the cage may help with ambulation. Soiling of the perineum may indicate an inability to self-clean. Rats should also be monitored to ensure they are able to urinate and defecate. If they are unable to move the tail well, there may be trauma and subsequent infection and necrosis.

INFECTIOUS DISEASE

The primary infectious disease of concern in the aged pet rat is murine respiratory mycoplasmosis (MRM), the major component of chronic respiratory disease. The causative agent is *Mycoplasma pulmonis*.[32] The infection is generally silent in young animals. Clinical signs in aged rats may include dyspnea, snuffling, chattering, rales, nasal discharge, chromodacryorrhea, and head tilt. Rats with severe middle-ear involvement may spin when suspended by the tail. The disease may be transmitted horizontally by aerosol and direct contact, and vertically in utero.[33] Venereal transmission may be possible. Mycoplasmosis should be differentiated from other bacterial pneumonias (such as cilia-associated respiratory bacillus, *Corynebacterium kutscheri,* and streptococcosis) and from viral mycotic and environmental causes. Mycoplasma may be cultured from exudate in the upper respiratory tract and middle ears.[3,6] Enrofloxacin (10 mg/kg by mouth every 12 hours) combined with doxycycline (5 mg/kg by mouth every 12 hours) have proven efficacious in treatment of MRM.[9]

TUMORS

Mammary tumors are common in older female rats. Of these mammary tumors 80% to 90% are benign fibroadenomas; the remainder are carcinomas. Genetic susceptibility is the most significant factor, although diet and environment may also play a role. Unlike in the mouse, retroviruses do not seem to play a role in development of mammary tumors in rats. Prolactin levels in rats with tumors have been reported to be 25 times higher than virgin females. These tumors may become large and infiltrate locally without metastasis. These tumors may be resected if not too large, but may recur in another mammary gland.[3,6]

Interstitial cell tumors have a high predominance in the males of some strains of rats (see earlier discussion). The testes may be removed surgically.

Pituitary adenoma is a common tumor in aged male and female rats. As with other tumors, genetic factors and diet may play a role. Rats may be asymptomatic or display profound depression and incoordination. It has been suggested that prolactin-producing pituitary tumors may be associated with increased incidence of mammary fibroadenomas.[34]

Large granular lymphocytic leukemia is a major cause of death in some strains of geriatric laboratory rats. Leukocyte counts of $400,000/mL^3$ have been seen. Enlarged spleen (which may be palpable), icterus, anemia, weight loss, and depression are characteristic clinical signs.[6,35]

GENERAL HUSBANDRY CONSIDERATIONS IN AGED RATS

The aged rat may have difficulty ambulating because of arthritic, neurologic, or muscular disease. The primary enclosure of these animals should allow for easy access to food and water. Toenails may become overgrown in smooth-bottomed cages and may be a particular problem in aged rats with altered stance and gait caused by arthritis or neuromuscular degeneration. Flooring and bedding should allow adequate traction. Increased urination secondary to renal disease may require more absorbent materials to be used and more frequent cleaning schedules. Compromised animals may have difficulty in maintaining body temperature. Additional bedding material and supplemental heat sources may be necessary. Caution should be taken not to overheat the rat. Heat lamps and heating pads pose greater risks than warm air or water blankets.

Medicating rats can be challenging although sweet medications such as pediatric amoxicillin drops are generally well accepted. Water should be medicated with caution. Rats may avoid drinking medicated water and this risks adequate hydration and inadequate dosing. Mixing a sweet juice with the water may increase palatability. Parental medication, oral medications hidden in sweet food or administered by gavage may be preferred. Flavored medicated rat treats are available commercially for the research arena.

If abdominal or lengthy surgery is necessary in the aged rat, inhalant anesthesia such as isoflurane generally yields a more stable plane of anesthesia than injectable rodent cocktails. Anesthesia methods, sedation, and anesthetic dosages are available in several publications.[9,10,36–40]

Diet and longevity studies in laboratory rats have indicated that caloric intake may be the single greatest influence on the incidence and severity of lesions and longevity.[11,12,19,41] High levels of dietary protein (22% or higher) are associated with a high incidence of chronic nephritis and diets comprised of 20% fat rather than 5% to 10% are life shortening. Additionally, protein over- and undernutrition have been shown to modify neoplasm incidence.[8,42]

SUMMARY

Geriatric disease in the pet rat is a sequela to aging, environment, and genetics and is not generally "curable." At best, the clinician may be able to offer improved quality of remaining life for some patients. The informed clinician, however, may be armed with sufficient information to help the owner of a geriatric rat understand the geriatric disease processes and make an informed decision on humane care for their pet, including selection of euthanasia when treatment options are limited, not effective, or not available.

Biomedical research continues to find new therapies aimed at improving the longevity and quality of life for humans and animals. The rat is central to this research. Research in the rat has included regeneration of spinal cord nerves and brain neurons, new pharmaceutical and gene therapy for heart failure, new treatments for chronic renal failure and organ transplantation.[43–45] The laboratory rat is often the first species in which proof of concept, dosing, and efficacy is verified. Pet rat medicine has the opportunity to access cutting-edge therapies for the companion rat, developed first in and for the rat.

REFERENCES

1. AVMA. Market research statistics. U.S. pet ownership & demographics sourcebook. Schaumburg (IL): American Veterinary Medicine Association; 2001.

2. AVMA. Market research statistics. U.S. pet ownership & demographics source-book. Schaumburg (IL): American Veterinary Medicine Association; 2007.
3. Kohn DF, Clifford CB. Biology and disease of rats. In: Fox JG, Anderson LC, Loew FM, et al, editors. Laboratory animal medicine. 2nd edition. New York: Academic Press; 2002. p. 121–65.
4. Davaiu J. Clinical evaluation of rodents. Veterinary Clin North Am Exot Anim Pract 1999;2(2):429–45.
5. Bivin WS, Crawford M, Brewer NR. Morphophysiology. In: Baker HJ, Lindsey JR, Weisbroth SH, editors. The laboratory rat, vol. 1. 1st edition. New York: Academic Press; 1979. p. 74–103.
6. Percy DH, Barthold SW. Rat. In: Pathology of laboratory rodents & rabbits. 2nd edition. Ames (IA): Iowa State University Press; 2001. p. 107–58.
7. Gray JE, Weaver RN, Purmalis A. Ultrastructural observations of chronic progressive nephrosis in the Sprague-Dawley rat. Vet Pathol 1974;11:153–64.
8. Anver MR, Cohen BJ. Lesions associated with aging. In: Baker HJ, Lindsey JR, Weisbroth SH, editors. The laboratory rat, vol. 1. 1st edition. New York: Academic Press; 1979. p. 378–99.
9. Rodents. In: Carpenter JW, editor. Exotic animal formulary. 3rd edition. St Louis (MO): Elsevier Inc; 2005. p. 376–408.
10. Hawk CT, Leary SL, Morris TH, in association with the American College of Laboratory Animal Medicine. Formulary for laboratory animals. 3rd edition. Ames (IA): Blackwell Publishing; 2005. p.163, 171.
11. Keenan KP, Soper KA, Hertzog PR, et al. Diet, overfeeding, and moderate dietary restriction in control Sprague-Dawley rats: 2. Effects on age-related proliferative and degenerative lesions. Toxicol Pathol 1995;23:287–302.
12. Gumprecht LA, Long CR, Soper KA, et al. The early effects of dietary restriction on the pathogenesis of chronic renal disease in Sprague-Dawley rats at 12 months. Toxicol Pathol 1993;21:528–37.
13. Leenen FD, Skarda V, Yuan B, et al. Changes in cardiac ANGII post myocardial infarction in rats: effects of nephrectomy and ACE inhibitors. Am J Phsyiol Heart Circ Physiol 1999;276:317–25.
14. Patterson M. Urolithiasis in the Sprague-Dawley rat. Lab Anim 1979;13:17–20.
15. Ekstrom ME, Ewald PE. Chronic purulent preputial gland adenitis in the male laboratory rat. Am Assoc Lab Anim Sci. Joilet, Illinois, 1975. Abstr no 10; Publ 75–2.
16. Franks LM. Normal and pathological anatomy and histology of the genital tract of rats and mice. In: Cotchin E, Roe FJ, editors. Pathology of laboratory rats and mice. Philadelphia: Davis; 1967. p. 469–99.
17. Wolfe JM, Burack E, Lensing W, et al. The effects of advancing age on the connective tissue of the uterus, cervix and vagina of the rat. Am J Anat 1942; 70:135–65.
18. Jenkins JR. Surgical sterilization in small mammals. Veterinary Clin North Am Exot Anim Pract 2000;3(3):617–27.
19. Keenan KP, Soper KA, Smith PF, et al. Diet, overfeeding and moderate dietary restriction in control Sprague-Dawley rats: 1. Effects on spontaneous neoplasms. Toxicol Pathol 1995;23:269–86.
20. Brower GL, Levick SP, Janicki JS. Inhibition of matrix metalloproteinase activity by ACE inhibitors prevents left ventricular remodeling in a rat model of heart failure. Am J Physiol Heart Circ Physiol 2007;292:3057–64.
21. Wohlgemuth SE, Julian D, Akin DE, et al. Autophagy in the heart and liver during normal aging and calorie restriction. Rejuvenation Res 2007;10:281–92.

22. Elwell MR, Stedham MA, Kovatch RM. In: Boorman GA, Eustis MR, Elwell CA, et al, editors. Pathology of the Fischer rat: reference and atlas. San Diego (CA): Academic Press; 1990. p. 261–77.
23. Wexler BC. Spontaneous coronary arteriosclerosis in repeatedly bred male and female rats. Circ Res 1964;14:32–43.
24. Witt CJ, Johnson LK. Diagnostic exercise: rear limb ataxia in a rat. Lab Anim Sci 1990;40:528–9.
25. Krinke GJ. Spontaneous radioneuropathology, aged rats. In: Jones TC, Mohr U, Hunt RD, et al, editors. Monographs on pathology of laboratory animals: nervous system. New York: Springer-Verlag; 1988. p. 203–8.
26. Medina-Santillan R, Reyes-Garcia G, Rocha-Gonzalez HI, et al. B vitamins increase the analgesic effect of ketorolac in the formalin test in the rat. Proc West Pharmacol Soc 2004;47:95–9.
27. Jolivalt CG, Mizisin LM, Nelson A, et al. B vitamins alleviate indices of neuropathic pain in diabetic rats. Eur J Pharmacol 2009;612(1–3):41–7.
28. Song XS, Huang ZJ, Song XJ. Thiamine suppresses thermal hyperalgesia, inhibits hyperexcitability and lessens alterations of sodium currents in injured, dorsal root ganglion neurons in rats. Anesthesiology 2009;110(2):387–400.
29. Van Steenis G, Kroes R. Changes in the nervous system and musculature of old rats. Vet Pathol 1971;8:320–32.
30. Marzettie E, Carter CS, Wohlgemuth SE, et al. Changes in IL-15 expression and death-receptor apoptotic signaling in rat gastrocnemius muscle with aging and life-long calorie restriction. Mech Ageing Dev 2009;130(4):272–80.
31. Pollard M, Kajima J. Lesions in aged germfree Wistar rats. Am J Pathol 1970;61: 25–32.
32. Kohn DF, Kirk BE. Pathogenicity of *Mycoplasma pulmonis* in laboratory rats. Lab Anim Care 1969;19:321–30.
33. Lindsey JR, Baker HJ, Overcash RG, et al. Murine chronic respiratory disease: significance as a research complication and experimental production with *Mycoplasma pulmonis*. Am J Pathol 1971;64:675–716.
34. Sandusky GE, Van Pelt CS, Todd GC, et al. An immunocytochemical study of pituitary adenoma and focal hyperplasia in old Sprague-Dawley and Fischer 344 rats. Toxicol Pathol 1988;16(3):376–80.
35. Rosol TJ, Stromberg PC. Effects of large granular lymphocytic leukemia on bone in F344 rats. Vet Pathol 1990;27:397–403.
36. Adamcak A, Otten B. Rodent therapeutics. Veterinary Clin North Am Exot Anim Pract 2000;3(1):221–38.
37. Yale Animal Resources Center. Comparative medicine. Vet Clin Serv Drugs Dosages 2009;1–4.
38. Wixon SK, Smiler KL. Anesthesia and analgesia in rodents. In: Kohn DF, Wixson SK, White WJ, et al, editors. Anesthesia and analgesia in laboratory animals. 1st edition. New York: Academic Press; 1997. p. 165–204.
39. Flecknell PA. Laboratory animal anesthesia. A practical introduction for research workers and technicians. San Diego (CA): Academic Press; 1996.
40. Cantwell SL. Ferret, rabbit and rodent anesthesia. Veterinary Clin North Am Exot Anim Pract 2001;4(1):169–91.
41. Anver MR, Cohen BJ. Nutrition. In: Baker HJ, Lindsey JR, Weisbroth SH, editors. The laboratory rat, vol. 1. 1st edition. New York: Academic Press; 1979. p. 123–52.
42. Ross MH, Bras G. Influence of protein under- and over-nutrition on spontaneous tumor prevalence in the rat. J Nutr 1973;103:944–63.

43. Gage FH, Dunnett SB, Stenevi U, et al. Aged rats: recovery of motor impairments by intrastriatal nigral grafts. Science 1983;221:966–9.
44. Carter CS, Leeuwenburgh CL, Daniels M, et al. Influence of calorie restriction on measures of age-related cognitive decline: role of increased physical activity. J Gerontol A Biol Sci Med Sci 2009;64(8):850–9.
45. Thomas Jefferson University. Gene therapy reversed heart damage in rats with heart failure. Science Daily. December 31, 2008.

The Senior Ferret (*Mustela Putorius Furo*)

Sharman M. Hoppes, DVM, DABVP-Avian

KEYWORDS

- Ferret • Geriatric • Neoplasia • Adrenal disease
- Lymphoma • Cardiomyopathy

Ferrets are an increasingly popular pet in the United States. They are active, gregarious pets that delight their owners with their playful antics. One of the issues that ferret owners and veterinarians have had to deal with is their shortened life span brought on by multiple disease processes. Although literature cites the life span of the ferret as 8 to 10 years of age, most exotic veterinarians routinely see ferrets as "old" at as early as 3 years of age. The majority of the information on senior ferrets has focused on neoplastic diseases, primarily adrenal tumors and insulinomas. This article discusses husbandry and nutritional issues of the aging ferret along with some of the more commonly seen geriatric diseases, including neoplasia, and the available diagnostics and treatment options.

Ferrets *(Mustela putorius furo)* have become a popular pet in the past decade. They belong to the family, Mustelidae, and are related to mink, martens, badgers, otters, and skunks. In the United Kingdom, ferrets were used for rodent control and hunting rabbits. These practices still occur in Europe but to a lesser degree. In the United States, ferrets have been used in research and as pets. Hunting with ferrets is illegal in the United States and ferrets are considered a companion animal. Most ferret owners are as committed to their ferrets as dog and cat owners are to their pets, and they seek the same veterinary care that others expect for their dogs and cats.

HUSBANDRY

Ferrets of all ages are curious active creatures and should be confined to a large cage or enclosure when not under close supervision, but they should not be caged 24 hours a day. They need time out of the cage for exercise and mental stimulation. Ferrets should be allowed to play in a ferret-proof area for several hours daily, and this time can be divided throughout the day. In their cage, ferrets should have a retreat for sleeping, in the form of a cloth tube, hammock, or tent. Ferrets can be trained to use a litter box—a corner box works well because they like to back up into corners to defecate. Litter boxes should be close and easily accessed, as ferrets have a short

Department of Veterinary Small Animal Sciences, Texas A&M University, College of Veterinary Medicine, 4474 TAMU, College Station, TX 77843-4474, USA
E-mail address: shoppes@cvm.tamu.edu

Vet Clin Exot Anim 13 (2010) 107–122
doi:10.1016/j.cvex.2009.12.002
1094-9194/10/$ – see front matter © 2010 Elsevier Inc. All rights reserved.

gastrointestinal transit time and may not make it to a litter box in another room or area of the house.

As ferrets age, some changes in their housing may be required. They may develop vision difficulties or they may not be as agile as they once were. Providing fewer levels for climbing, adjusting ramps so they are easier to climb, placing shelves closer together, and making sure food and water bowls are accessible may be necessary. For some elderly ferrets affected by multiple diseases, a smaller one-story cage may be safer.

Ferrets are predatory hunters and should be monitored closely when housed with other pets, especially other pocket pets, birds, or reptiles. This is true even with older ferrets. They are extremely playful and play hard for hours followed by a long nap. Senior ferrets often play less and sleep more, and with advancing age many ferrets sleep the majority of the day and night.

DIET

Ferrets are strict carnivores. They have a short gastrointestinal tract that empties in 3 to 4 hours. Due to diminished gastrointestinal flora and few brush border enzymes, they do not metabolize carbohydrates well.[1] They also have difficulty digesting fiber. They require diets high in good-quality animal protein and fat with minimal carbohydrates and fiber. Excess carbohydrates may lead to pancreatic disease, such as insulinoma. Treats that are acceptable include pieces of chicken, eggs, and other high-protein snacks. Ferrets develop their dietary preferences in the first few months of age, so it is important that they be started on an appropriate diet early.[1] Changing an adult or older ferret's diet can be challenging. A whole prey diet has been advocated by many authorities and is fed in some areas of the world. In the United States, a good-quality dry ferret or kitten diet is recommended to aid in prevention of dental disease. As ferrets age, a switch to a senior ferret diet should be considered. Several geriatric diets are available. Weight loss, emaciation, and muscle wasting can occur in older ferrets. Long-term anorexia can lead to hepatic lipidosis. More frequent feedings and assisted feedings may be necessary in sick or senior ferrets (**Fig. 1**).

VETERINARY CARE

The literature reports that the life span of ferrets can be up to 10 years of age, but most ferrets in North America live 5 to 7 years, with the onset of many geriatric and

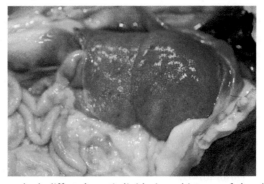

Fig. 1. Ferret with marked, diffuse hepatic lipidosis and icterus of the abdominal adipose. (*Courtesy of* C.M. Pfent.)

neoplastic diseases seen as early as 3 years of age.[2] Most exotic veterinarians consider ferrets "senior" at 3 to 4 years of age. At this age it is recommended that ferrets have physical examinations performed twice a year and yearly blood work. Blood work may include complete blood count (CBC), chemistry profile, and possibly an adrenal panel, depending on the age and health of a ferret. With many disease processes, CBC and chemistry profiles may need to be performed more frequently.

FERRET RESTRAINT AND PHYSICAL EXAMINATION

Ferrets of any age are typically easily restrained for physical examination. Most ferrets tolerate gentle restraint on a table. If a ferret is difficult to restrain or fractious, scruffing a ferret at the back of its neck and suspending it off the table results in relaxation and allows for physical examination.[3]

VENIPUNCTURE

Venipuncture sites for ferrets include the jugular vein, cranial vena cava, and cephalic and lateral saphenous. Many ferrets can be restrained for venipuncture without sedation or anesthesia. For jugular venipuncture, the technique used in cats, with head tilted back and forelegs pulled forward over the edge of a table, works well. The jugular vein in ferrets is slightly more lateral than in cats or dogs. For the cranial vena cava approach, a ferret is held on its back with its front legs pulled caudally and the head and neck extended. A 25-gauge needle is inserted into the thoracic cavity between the manubrium and first rib at a 45° angle, pointing the needle toward the opposite rear leg. The needle is inserted to its hub, then slowly withdrawn while gently applying suction until blood begins to fill the syringe. For difficult or fractious ferrets, the author routinely masks them down with isoflurane or sevoflurane briefly to obtain the sample. Isoflurane anesthesia can reduce the hematocrit level, red blood cell count, and hemoglobin concentrations so be sure to note that the sample is taken with the ferret under anesthesia in the evaluation of the blood sample.[4]

PREVENTIVE CARE

Preventive medicine for older ferrets includes yearly to twice-a-year physical examinations, distemper and rabies vaccination, monthly heartworm preventative, and dental prophylaxis. Ferrets of all ages are susceptible to canine distemper, which is a fatal disease in ferrets. PureVax (Merial, Athens, Georgia) is the distemper vaccine recommended for ferrets.[5] Vaccination for rabies is also recommend and required in some states. The Imrab 3 (Merial, Athens, GA, USA) killed vaccine is approved for use in ferrets.[6]

Ferrets are susceptible to vaccine reactions.[7] Mild reactions may include pruritis or weakness. More severe reactions include vomiting, diarrhea, hyperthermia, or, rarely, death. The author routinely premedicates ferrets with diphenhydramine (2 mg/kg subcutaneously 20 minutes before vaccination) and then monitors ferrets for a minimum of 30 minutes post vaccination. In older ferrets with multiple diseases present and any history of vaccine reaction, it is important to weigh the benefits and risks of vaccination.

Vaccine injection–site sarcomas have also been documented in ferrets, although no particular vaccine was identified as the culprit.[8] Implementing the vaccine protocols used in cats may be prudent.

Ferrets are susceptible to heartworm disease and should be on a monthly preventative in endemic areas. Recommended monthly preventatives include selamectin, applied topically (6 mg/kg); ivermectin (0.05 mg/kg by mouth or subcutaneously); or milbemycin oxime (1.15 to 2.33 mg/kg by mouth).[9]

COMMON GERIATRIC DISEASES

Ferrets are well known for the development of several geriatric disorders. They have a high incidence of tumors, with neoplasia often the cause of or a contributing factor to death in geriatric ferrets. Gastrointestinal disease, dental disease, cardiomyopathy, renal disease, and cataracts are other common diseases in senior ferrets.

GASTROINTESTINAL DISEASE

Gastrointestinal disease occurs commonly in older ferrets, with trichobezoars, gastric ulcers, epizootic catarrhal enteritis, and inflammatory bowel disease the most commonly reported causes.[10,11]

Although foreign bodies are the most common cause of gastrointestinal obstruction in young ferrets, in older ferrets trichobezoars are a more common cause.[12] Clinical signs of obstruction include anorexia, lethargy, hypersalivation, and pain on abdominal palpation. Vomiting occurs infrequently in ferrets but if present is supportive of obstructive disease. Weight loss can be significant if the obstruction is chronic. Abdominal radiographs may reveal a fluid- or gas-filled stomach and a gas pattern in the intestinal tract. The trichobezoar may or may not be radiographically evident. Medical therapy includes fluid therapy and laxatone, but in many cases surgery is necessary.

Gastric ulcers can occur in young and old ferrets. Gastrointestinal ulcers are often secondary to other disease processes, such as gastrointestinal neoplasia, foreign body, drug therapy, renal disease, or *Helicobacter mustelae* infection.[10,11] Clinical signs of gastric ulcers include lethargy, ptyalism, diarrhea, teeth grinding, melena, and pain on abdominal palpation. A presumptive diagnosis can be reached through the use of diagnostics, including radiographs, CBC and biochemical profile, biopsy, or response to treatment. CBC may reveal a mild to moderate regenerative anemia. A definitive diagnosis can be reached with endoscopy. *H mustelae* infections can be difficult to diagnose as it is believed that most ferrets are infected, so presence of the organism is not definitive for disease. Treatment options include treating any underlying disease in conjunction with treatment of the gastric ulcers. For treatment of gastric ulcers, a combination of amoxicillin (20 mg/kg by mouth every 12 h) and metronidazole (20 mg/kg by mouth every 12 h) is recommended along with systemic H_2-receptor antagonists: ranitidine (24 mg/kg every 8 h), famotidine (0.5 mg/kg by mouth every 24 h), or cimetidine (10 mg/kg every 8 h).[9,10] Depending on the severity of the disease, supportive care may be necessary.

Epizootic catarrhal enteritis is a highly contagious disease caused by a coronavirus that can spread rapidly through a collection of ferrets.[10,11] The history often includes the addition of a young ferret to a home with older ferrets. The young ferret is often clinically normal, but the older ferrets in the home develop symptoms within a few days. Clinical signs include depression, lethargy, watery green diarrhea, melena, dehydration, and weight loss. Diagnostics include CBC, biochemical profile, and radiographs. CBC may reveal a leukocytosis, a monocytosis, and a mild to severe anemia. Serum urea nitrogen, alanine aminotransferase (ALT), and alkaline phosphatase may be elevated. Radiographs may reveal ileus. Supportive care includes aggressive fluid therapy, antibiotics, and nutritional support. All affected ferrets should be isolated.

Inflammatory bowel disease is common in older ferrets.[13] This disease is typically multifactorial in ferrets. A chronic form of coronavirus (epizootic catarrhal enteritis) has been reported as a causative agent, as has *H mustelae* infection. Other suspected causes include dietary intolerance or hypersensitivity. A history of previous illness with epizootic catarrhal enteritis, along with chronic loose birdseed-like stools, may aid in the diagnosis of inflammatory bowel disease, but full-thickness gastric and intestinal biopsies are necessary for a definitive diagnosis.[10] Histopathology may reveal a lymphoplasmacytic or eosinophilic inflammation. Treatments include dietary management often with a hypoallergenic diet, prednisone (1 mg/kg by mouth every 12 h), or azathioprine (0.9 mg/kg by mouth every 24 to 72 h).[9]

A recent study performed at Texas A&M University revealed that ferrets, similarly to cats, have diminished cobalamin levels when afflicted with chronic diarrhea.[14] This study revealed that ferrets with chronic diarrhea have significantly decreased serum concentrations of cobalamin, and significantly increased serum concentrations of methylmalonic acid. These findings suggest that cobalamin malabsorption is common in ferrets with chronic diarrhea and that it can be severe enough to cause increases in serum methylmalonic acid concentrations indicating tissue depletion of cobalamin. Although only a few ferrets have been followed after cobalamin therapy, the preliminary results suggest that cobalamin therapy is helpful in treatment of chronic diarrhea in ferrets.[14] The author's current recommendations are extrapolated from cobalamin therapy in cats: cobalamin (250 μg subcutaneously per ferret weekly for 6 weeks, then 250 μg every 2 weeks for 6 weeks, then monthly). Cobalamin levels should be re-evaluated 1 month after the last administration. Monthly injections may be necessary in chronic intestinal disease.[14]

NEOPLASIA

Adrenal tumors are one of the most common endocrine tumors in domestic ferrets.[15] Middle-aged to older ferrets are affected most often. The cause of adrenal tumors in ferrets is unknown; many theories have been considered. Early neutering has been implicated as have husbandry and nutrition issues. In the United States, ferrets are neutered at a few weeks of age, are housed indoors, and are on formulated diets. European ferrets are neutered later, often housed outdoors, and are fed a whole prey diet. A recent article revealed that when ferrets are neutered at a later age in Europe they too develop adrenal disease, indicating that it does not appear to be the age of neutering but the act of neutering that results in disease.[16]

In contrast to canine and human adrenal disease (Cushing disease), serum cortisol levels are not elevated.[17] In ferrets, one or more of the plasma hormones are elevated: estradiol, 17-hydroxyprogesterone, or androstenedione. These elevations can occur with adrenal cortical hyperplasia, adenoma, or adenocarcinoma.[17]

Bilateral progressive alopecia, often accompanied by pruritus, is the most commonly reported clinical sign. Hair loss occurs in both genders and typically progresses from the tail forward to the shoulders and neck. Female ferrets may have an enlarged vulva and male ferrets an enlarged prostate.[15] Male ferrets may present with stranguria secondary to prostatic hyperplasia or prostatic cysts. Severe prostatomegaly can lead to urinary obstruction and result in acute renal failure.[18] Affected male ferrets may also exhibit aggression.

If significantly enlarged, the adrenal gland may be palpable. The left adrenal is located in a large fat pad cranial to the left kidney. The right adrenal is cranial to the right kidney and beneath a lobe of the liver, making it more difficult to palpate even if enlarged (**Fig. 2**).

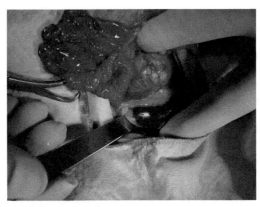

Fig. 2. Grossly enlarged left adrenal gland in a ferret.

A presumptive diagnosis of adrenal cortical tumors in domestic ferrets can be reached based on history and clinical signs. CBC values are usually within normal limits. Occasionally, an anemia may be present, and in severe cases a pancytopenia similar to that seen as a result of estrogen toxicity may be seen. A packed cell volume of less than 15% is associated with a grave prognosis. The serum chemistry profile is usually within normal limits, although ALT may be elevated. Radiographs can be helpful in reaching a presumptive diagnosis if an adrenal tumor is large enough to be visible or if there is displacement of other organs. Ultrasound can be used to determine the size and extent of tumors in association with other structures, such as the liver or caudal vena cava.[17]

The dexamethasone suppression test and adrenocorticotropic hormone stimulation test are not useful as cortisol levels are not elevated.[17] A definitive diagnosis of adrenal cortical tumors can be reached by measuring plasma hormone levels or histopathology. A hormone plasma steroid panel measuring estradiol, 17-hydroxyprogesterone, or androstenedione is offered by the University of Tennessee.[19]

Treatment includes medical and surgical options. Surgery consists of adrenalectomy and may be preferred if a ferret is in otherwise good health.[15] CBC, chemistry profile, radiographs, and ultrasound should be performed before surgery. A thorough abdominal exploratory should be performed with evaluation of both adrenal glands and excision of the affected gland. If both adrenal glands are affected, bilateral adrenalectomy is recommended. The right adrenal gland is adjacent to the caudal vena cava and when enlarged may invade the vena cava. Because of this close proximity or invasion into the caudal vena cava, complete excision of the right adrenal gland is often not possible. Reoccurrence may take place in the remaining adrenal gland or in any residual tissue left after a right adrenalectomy.[18] Male ferrets with prostatomegaly or prostatic cysts should have the prostatic cysts drained and marsupialized.[17] Whenever surgery is performed on a ferret, evaluation of the gastrointestinal tract, spleen, lymph nodes, kidney, and pancreas should be included.

The medical approach is often chosen in older ferrets with concurrent diseases or ferrets that are poor anesthetic and surgical candidates. Drugs commonly used in the treatment of adrenal tumors of ferrets include leuprolide, anastrozole, and melatonin. Less commonly used drugs include flutamide and bicalutamide.

Leuprolide acetate (Lupron) is a gonadotropin-releasing hormone analog (GnRH) and is one of the most widely used drugs for adrenal tumors in ferrets.[20] Although Lupron aids in the reduction of clinical signs, there is usually not a reduction in the size of the affected adrenal gland. In studies on Lupron and its affects on ferrets with adrenal tumors, Lupron eliminated the clinical signs and reduced the concentrations of the affected sex hormones.[20] The recommended dosage is 100 to 500 μg/kg intramuscularly or subcutaneously every 3 to 8 weeks. Dosage and interval vary depending on individuals. Most ferrets need to be treated for the rest of their lives.

Melatonin implants have been successful in stimulating hair growth. Melatonin has been used for years to stimulate molt and winter coat growth in farmed minks. The exact mechanism of action is unknown. It is thought to aid in regulation of GnRH secretion through specific receptors in the pituitary and hypothalamus, negatively affecting GnRH secretion, decreasing LH and FSH, and ultimately reducing sex hormones. Studies have revealed reduction of plasma steroids, dramatic regrowth of hair, and reduction of vulvar swelling or prostatic size.[21]

Other drugs that have been used to treat adrenal disease in ferrets include anastrozole (Arimidex), an aromatase inhibitor that lowers estrogen by converting adrenal-generated androstenedione to estrone by aromatase in peripheral tissues[22]; flutamide (Eulexin), which inhibits androgen uptake and binding in target tissues[15]; and bicalutamide (Casodex), which competitively inhibits the action of androgens at the receptor site.[22] Flutamide and bicalutamide have been used in ferrets to reduce the size of prostatic tissue and diminish clinical signs of adrenal disease.[15,22]

INSULINOMA

Pancreatic islet cell tumors are one of the most common tumors in middle-aged and older ferrets. Beta cell tumors or insulinomas are the most frequently diagnosed islet cell tumor in ferrets.[23,24] Reported age for ferrets with insulinoma ranges from 2 to 7 years with an average of 5 years.[25] Pancreatic islet cell tumors produce insulin, resulting in increased insulin secretion and subsequent hypoglycemia. Male and female ferrets are affected.

The history may include a ferret that is "sleeping more." Clinical signs may vary immensely, from asymptomatic ferrets with hypoglycemia detected on routine hematology to ferrets presenting with weakness, ataxia, posterior paresis, hypersalivation, and seizuring (**Fig. 3**).

Diagnosis is based on a documented hypoglycemia. A blood glucose level of less than 60 mg/dL is diagnostic. History and clinical signs are usually supportive of the diagnosis.[15] Hematology and chemistry profiles are often unremarkable as are radiographs. Ultrasound may pick up large pancreatic nodules but often small discrete insulinomas are undetectable (**Fig. 4**).

Treatment options include surgical excision and medical management.[15] Medical management may reduce clinical signs of disease but does not stop progression of the tumor. Dietary recommendations include a meat-based, high-protein ferret or

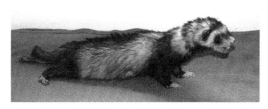

Fig. 3. Hindlimb paresis in a geriatric ferret with insulinoma. (*Courtesy of* C.M. Pfent.)

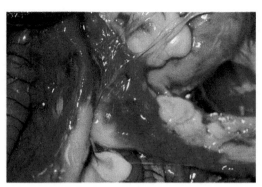

Fig. 4. Pancreatic islet cell adenomas (insulinomas) are often multiple and less than 2 mm in size. This 6-mm insulinoma is easier to identify at surgery or necropsy. (*Courtesy of* C.M. Pfent.)

cat food with high-protein treats, such as chicken, egg, or chicken- or liver-flavored feline treats. High-sugar or high-carbohydrate treats should be avoided. Food should be available at all times. Severely affected ferrets may require additional feedings at night to avoid a hypoglycemic crisis. Owners should be instructed on identifying early signs of hypoglycemia and to have honey or corn syrup available for an acute crisis.

Drug therapy includes prednisone or prednisolone and diazoxide used singly or in combination. Prednisone or prednisolone increases peripheral blood glucose concentrations by inhibiting glucose uptake by peripheral tissues and increasing hepatic gluconeogenesis. Dosage may range from 0.25 mg/kg to 2 mg/kg every 12 hours.[9] Many ferrets can be managed medically with prednisone alone at least initially. With progression of the disease, increasing doses of prednisone are needed. Diazoxide is a benzothiadiazide diuretic that inhibits release of insulin from the beta cells, promotes gluconeogenesis, and decreases cellular uptake of glucose. Diazoxide should be added to the medical protocol when prednisone alone is no longer effective. The dosage for diazoxide is 10 to 30 mg/kg every 12 hours, beginning at the low end of the range and increasing the dose as needed.[9] Often the dose of prednisone can be reduced with the addition of diazoxide. Diazoxide is expensive and cost prohibitive for some owners.

Surgical therapy is the treatment of choice but is often not curative. One study reported 53% of ferrets still required medical management for hypoglycemia after surgery.[26] Surgery involves excision of all pancreatic nodules, if possible, or partial pancreatectomy, if indicated. Although most ferrets need medical therapy if not immediately then within months of surgery, it has been shown that ferrets with surgery have a longer survival time than those on medical therapy alone.[25] Another benefit to surgery is that even if medical therapy is required postoperatively, it is usually at a much reduced dosage. Blood glucose should be monitored 7 to 14 days postoperatively and then every 2 to 3 months. Prognosis for insulinoma is dependent on severity of disease, with reports of mean survival times of 668 days after surgery.[26] The age of a ferret and concurrent diseases can affect prognosis.

LYMPHOMA

The term, *lymphoma* or *lymphosarcoma*, refers to the invasion of any organ or lymph node with atypical lymphocytes. Lymphoma and lymphosarcoma are both used to describe malignant disease. Lymphoma is one of the most common neoplastic diseases in ferrets. It has been described in all ages and can affect most organs. It primarily affects the lymph nodes, mediastinal lymphatic tissue, and intestines. A viral etiology has been proposed but has not been validated.[27,28]

Lymphoma in ferrets is often broken down into two distinct syndromes: a juvenile form and an adult-onset form.[29] The juvenile form occurs in ferrets less than 2 years of age. The most common presentation is acute respiratory distress due to the presence of a cranial mediastinal mass. This is known as lymphoblastic lymphoma.

The adult form is seen in ferrets more than 3 years of age. Lymphadenopathy is often present. This is often termed *lymphocytic lymphoma*. This disease has a slower progression and more chronic pattern than the juvenile form.[18,29] Clinical signs vary according to organ system affected and include weakness, dyspnea, depression, anorexia, weight loss, diarrhea, and maldigestion.

Physical examination may reveal a weakened, thin, or emaciated ferret. There may be a peripheral lymphadenopathy. Hepatomegaly, splenomegaly, and thickened intestines may be palpable.

Diagnostics include a CBC, chemistry profile, radiographs, and ultrasound. Hematology may reveal a leukocytosis or leukopenia with or without a lymphocytosis. There may be elevations in liver or kidney enzymes reflecting organ involvement. Radiographs may reveal hepatomegaly, splenomegaly, mediastinal masses, or other masses in the thorax or abdomen. Ultrasound and ultrasound-guided fine-needle aspirates or biopsies with cytology or histopathology may be necessary for a definitive diagnosis.[30] Biopsy of a popliteal lymph node is recommended if there is a generalized peripheral lymphadenopathy. CT can aid in determining the presence of tumors. CT can provide excellent contrast between tissue types. The density of the mass can be compared with normal tissue to aid in determining size and invasiveness.[18] MRI is recommended if there is a suspicion of a tumor of the brain or spinal chord.[18]

In other species, a staging scheme has been developed to aid in determining proper treatment and prognosis. A classification scheme used in dogs has been accepted for ferrets.[18]

Stage 1: single site involvement (lymph node or other single site)
Stage 2: two or more noncontiguous sites on same side of diaphragm
Stage 3: multiple lymphatic sites on both sides of diaphragm (spleen, lymph node)
Stage 4: multiple sites on both sides of diaphragm, including nonlymphatic tissue or bone marrow involvement.

There are many treatment options for lymphoma available for several species. Several have been described in ferrets.[18] These chemotherapeutic protocols have been modified from canine and feline medicine.[18] Available treatment options often do not cure but only result in temporary remission. Surgery may be indicated for excision of tumors or affected organs. Chemotherapy includes treatment with prednisolone alone, which may result in rapid although temporary remission, to more aggressive chemotherapeutic protocols.

Many of the multimodal chemotherapeutic therapies involve frequent hospital visits, potentially caustic intravenous drugs and significant cost. The use of venous access ports is recommended to aid in the administration of frequent intravenous therapies.[18] Radiation treatment is also an available option for drug-resistant lymphomas or owners who do not feel comfortable with chemotherapy. Treatment goals should be discussed with the owner. Slowing down tumor growth, thereby extending or improving the quality of a ferret's life versus providing an actual cure, may be a realistic goal in most cases.

OTHER TUMORS

Other tumors that have been documented in ferrets include pancreatic adenocarcinoma, chordoma, chondrosarcoma, osteoma, thymoma, and hemangiosarcoma, which occurs most commonly in the liver and spleen. Hepatocellular and biliary adenocarcinomas and adenomas have also been reported.[23,24,29]

Ferrets have several types of cutaneous neoplasms, including basal cell tumors and mast cell tumors; both are usually benign and surgical excision is curative.[29]

CARDIOMYOPATHY

Cardiac disease is common in older ferrets.[31,32] Dilated and hypertrophic cardiomyopathy, valvular disease, and heartworm disease have all been documented. Dilated cardiomyopathy is the most common form of heart disease in domestic ferrets.[31] The cause of dilated cardiomyopathy in ferrets is unknown. The cause in cats has been linked to a deficiency in taurine, and in dogs there is a genetic component, but the effect of diet or genetics in ferrets is undetermined. Hypertrophic cardiomyopathy also occurs but not as commonly. It is important to distinguish between the two disease processes for proper treatment.

Dilated cardiomyopathy usually occurs in ferrets over 3 years of age.[31] There is no sex predilection. The clinical signs include lethargy, weight loss, anorexia, coughing, distended abdomen, and exercise intolerance.[31] Cardiac disease is often not diagnosed early in older ferrets because owners often attribute the lethargy or "sleeping a lot" to age.

Left-sided heart murmurs may be auscultated, and often a tachycardia (350 to 400 bpm) is present.[31,32] Biochemical and hematologic parameters are often normal. Electrocardiographically, there may not be changes. Sinus tachycardia and ventricular and atrial premature complexes may be detected. Radiographically, an enlarged globoid heart may be noted, and this could be indicative of actual cardiac enlargement or pericardial effusion.[33] An elevated trachea or increased sternal contact of the heart may be seen. Other radiographic signs include ascites, hepatomegaly, splenomegaly, or pulmonary edema.[33]

Ultrasound is necessary for definitive diagnosis. Ultrasound distinguishes between hypertrophic and dilated cardiomyopathy, pleural and pericardial effusion, and heartworm disease and thoracic masses.[33] Definitive diagnosis is critical for therapy.

Treatment for heart disease in ferrets is similar to treatment in dogs and cats. Oxygen therapy should be initiated in dyspneic ferrets. Furosemide is given initially at 2.2 mg/kg every 8 to 12 hours. With dilated cardiomyopathy, digoxin (0.01 mg/kg every 24 h) may be initiated. Enalapril (0.25 to 0.5 mg/kg every 48 h) or captopril (one-eighth of a 12.5-mg tablet by mouth every 48 h) may be added if no renal disease is present. Nitroglycerin ointment may be used on initial presentation as a vasodilator by applying one-eighth of an inch strip to the inner pinna every 12 to 24 hours.[31,33] Pimobendan may be used (0.5 mg/kg by mouth every 12 h) for dilated cardiomyopathy or valvular disease.[33]

Hypertrophic cardiomyopathy is rarer but does occur.[33] Oxygen therapy may be warranted along with diuretics, such as furosemide; β-blockers, such as atenolol (3 to 6 mg by mouth every 24 h); or a calcium channel blocker, such as diltiazem (1.75 to 7.5 mg by mouth every 12 h).[33]

Ferrets are susceptible to heartworm disease and this should be considered when clinical signs of heart disease are present in endemic areas. Heartworm disease in ferrets produces low numbers of microfilaria and, therefore, microfilarial testing can be unrewarding. ELISA-based antigen tests may be effective but with low worm burdens false-negative results may occur.[31] Ultrasound is often the best diagnostic tool allowing visualization of the worms.[34] There are few treatment options available for heartworm disease in ferrets. Ultrasound-guided retrieval of heartworms has been performed successfully at Texas A&M University. Treatments include steroids to reduce inflammation, ivermectin therapy, and cage rest. Ferrets in endemic areas should be on heartworm preventative.

RENAL DISEASE

Clinical illness due to renal disease is somewhat rare in ferrets, yet renal pathology is often seen on necropsy of older ferrets.[35,36] Many ferrets over the age of 4 years have varying degrees of chronic interstitial nephritis on necropsy. Early lesions may be seen in ferrets as young as 2 years of age. The disease is often progressive with pathologic changes that may or may not lead to renal failure, and the cause of death is infrequently related to kidney disease.[37,38] The most commonly reported pathologic changes in the kidneys of ferrets include interstitial nephritis and renal cysts.[35,36] Other causes of renal pathology include Aleutian mink disease, toxins, urolithiasis, and neoplasia **(Fig. 5)**.[18,36]

Renal cysts are common in ferrets, although their etiology is unknown. Most renal cysts are not a cause of renal disease and are an incidental finding during ultrasound examination, at surgery, or on necropsy **(Fig. 6)**.[38,39]

Aleutian mink disease is a parvovirus that often presents as a chronic wasting disease in ferrets. It can occur in ferrets of any age. Clinical signs include weight loss, depression, posterior paresis, and anemia. The disease results in a marked inflammatory response that can eventually lead to glomerulonephritis and marked interstitial nephritis, which results in renal failure and death.[39,40]

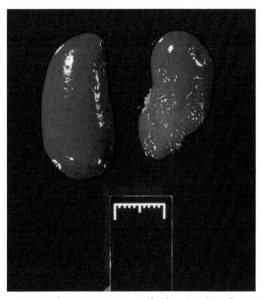

Fig. 5. Chronic interstitial nephritis is a common finding in older ferrets but is rarely problematic clinically. (*Courtesy of* C.M. Pfent.)

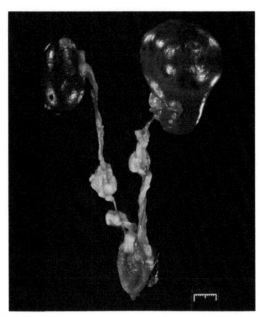

Fig. 6. Renal cysts in ferrets can range from 1 mm to several centimeters in size. Veterinarians should use caution not to mistake large benign renal cysts for hydronephrosis on ultrasound or by other imaging tools. (*Courtesy of* C.M. Pfent.)

Several toxicoses have been reported in ferrets, including zinc, copper, and ibuprofen. Ferrets of all ages should be monitored closely when not confined to their cages to avoid potential ingestion of toxins.[41–45]

Urolithiasis has been reported, but the incidence is reduced with the development of improved diets in ferrets.[37]

Clinical signs of renal disease in ferrets are similar to other companion animals and include depression, lethargy, weakness, posterior paresis, anorexia, weight loss, muscle wasting, and polyuria/polydipsia. Physical examination may reveal emaciation, dehydration, pale mucous membranes, and irregularly shaped kidneys.[38]

Initial diagnostics include a CBC, biochemical profile, and urinalysis. The biochemical profile may reveal hyperphosphatemia and elevated serum urea nitrogen. The creatinine in ferrets does not elevate markedly in renal disease.[35] In ferrets a creatinine of 2 mg/dL is significant. Other blood parameters that may be affected include an elevation in plasma proteins and a nonregenerative anemia. With plasma protein elevations, a protein electrophoresis or Aleutian disease testing should be submitted. Isosthenuria may be present on the urinalysis.[38]

Additional diagnostics include radiographs and ultrasound. Radiographs may reveal changes in kidney size or shape. Ultrasound can confirm changes and determine if renal architecture is normal. Ultrasound-guided biopsies or fine-needle aspirates may aid in reaching a definitive diagnosis.

Treatment in ferrets is similar to that of other mammals with renal disease. Fluid therapy can be administered intravenously in acute disease or subcutaneously by the owners at home in chronic cases. Antibiotics are included if infection is present, and phosphorus binders can be administered if indicated. Erythropoietin may aid in resolving nonregenerative anemia. The dosage for erythropoietin is 50 to 150 International Units subcutaneously 3 times a week until a desired packed cell volume is reached, then weekly.[9] Dietary changes can be challenging because ferrets are strict carnivores and require a high-protein diet.

DENTAL DISEASE

Dental calculi and fractured canines are the most common dental diseases in older ferrets.[11] A dry diet may decrease the incidence of calculi formation, which can lead to the development of gingivitis.[11,12] Yearly dental prophylaxis should be performed in older ferrets. Owners should be encouraged to provide dental care at home, including brushing teeth (**Fig. 7**).[12]

CATARACTS

Cataracts are the most common ophthalmic condition in ferrets. The cause is unknown, although genetics and dietary factors have been discussed as potential etiologies.[32] They can occasionally occur in young ferrets but more commonly occur in older ferrets. Because they progress slowly, ferrets adapt to diminished vision and owners may not readily notice anything and may even believe that acute blindness has occurred after a sudden change in a ferret's environment. Ferrets adapt well to cataract-induced blindness and manage well in home environments. Cataract surgery is an option, and phacoemulsification and extracapsular extraction have been performed successfully.[46]

SPLENOMEGALY

Splenomegaly is a common finding in older ferrets. There are several potential causes of splenomegaly, including neoplasia, hypersplenism, heart disease, and extramedullary hematopoiesis, the latter being the most common cause of splenomegaly in ferrets.[31] With extramedullary hematopoiesis, the spleen appears large but smooth in texture. Splenomegaly associated with lymphoma or other neoplastic processes is often nodular and white or tan nodules may be present.[47] Splenomegaly is often an incidental finding on physical examination, during ultrasound, or at surgery or necropsy. Often the spleen is large and easily palpated. If pathology is suspected, ultrasound-guided aspiration or aspiration through the abdominal wall can be performed relatively safely. Splenectomy should not be performed unless there is

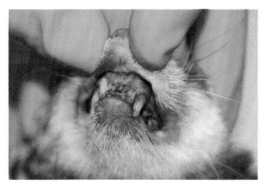

Fig. 7. Dental disease is common in geriatric ferrets. In this ferret, incisors 101, 201, 301, 302, 401, and 402 are missing and the canines 204 and 304 are fractured. The remaining teeth are covered with dental calculi. (*Courtesy of* C.M. Pfent.)

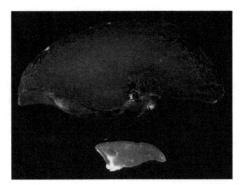

Fig. 8. The cross-section of a normal spleen is compared with markedly enlarged spleen diagnosed with extramedullary hematopoiesis. (*Courtesy of* J.F. Edwards and C.M. Pfent.)

documented pathology or the spleen has become so large it is impairing mobility of a ferret (**Fig. 8**).[47]

DEALING WITH LOSS

The emotional bond of owners to their ferrets is strong, similar to the bond owners develop with their dogs and cats. Clients have often spent many hours caring for their elderly pet, strengthening this bond even further. This can make euthanasia a difficult decision for owners. Determining when the time is right to euthanize can be challenging. Discussing the quality of life of ferrets is important in helping owners determine if that time has come. Is the pet able to get around on its own? Is it eating? Is the pet playful or able to enjoy interactions with the client? Are there more good days than bad? Often owners ask if it is better to allow a pet to die at home or be humanely euthanized. If the animal is not in pain or suffering and has an adequate quality of life, keeping the pet home and allowing it to die of "old age" may be an option. But often these animals have debilitating disease and may have multiple diseases present that are uncomfortable if not painful to the animal. It is veterinarians' responsibility to discuss with clients the option of euthanasia as an alternative to days or weeks of suffering. Euthanasia can be a painless, gentle end to a long, happy life for many pets. Owners can be allowed to be present with their pet. Presedation may be necessary in some pets, and placement of an intravenous catheter reduces stress for the client and the pet. If euthanasia is chosen, offering burial or cremation services is often appreciated by grieving owners, as are remembrance items, such as clay paws and locks of hair.

REFERENCES

1. Bell JA. Ferret nutrition. Vet Clin North Am Exotic Anim Pract 1999;2:169–92.
2. Brown S. Basic anatomy, physiology, and husbandry. In: Quesenberry KE, Carpenter JW, editors. Ferrets, rabbits and rodents: clinical medicine and surgery. 2nd edition. Philadelphia: WD Saunders; 2003. p. 2–12.
3. Quesenberry KE, Orcutt C. Basic approach to veterinary care. In: Quesenberry KE, Carpenter JW, editors. Ferrets, rabbits and rodents: clinical medicine and surgery. 2nd edition. Philadelphia: WD Saunders; 2003. p. 13–23.
4. Marini RP, Jackson LR, Esteves MI, et al. Effect of isoflurane on hematologic variables in ferrets. Am J Vet Res 1994;55:1479–83.

5. Tanner PA, Tseggai T, Rice Conlon JA, et al. Minimum protective dose (MPD) and efficacy determination of a recombinant canine distemper virus vaccine in ferrets. In: Proceedings of 81st Annual Meeting of the Conference of Research Workers in Animal Diseases. Chicago, November 12–14, 2000. Abstract 156.
6. Rupprecht CE, Gilbert J, Pitts R, et al. Evaluation of an inactivated rabies vaccine in domestic ferrets. J Am Vet Med Assoc 1990;196:1614–6.
7. Meyer EK. Vaccine associated adverse events. Vet Clin North Am Small Anim Pract 2001;31:494–514.
8. Munday JS, Stedman N, Richey LJ. Histology and immunochemistry of seven ferret vaccination-site fibrosarcomas. Vet Pathol 2003;40:288–93.
9. Carpenter JW, Mashima TY, Rupiper DJ. Exotic animal formulary. 2nd edition. Philadelphia: WB Saunders; 2001.
10. Jenkins J. Gastrointestinal diseases. In: Quesenberry KE, Carpenter JW, editors. Ferrets, rabbits and rodents: clinical medicine and surgery. 2nd edition. Philadelphia: WD Saunders; 2003. p. 161–71.
11. Fox JG. Diseases of the gastrointestinal system. In: Fox JG, editor. Biology and diseases of the ferret. Baltimore (MD): Williams & Wilkins; 1998. p. 273–90.
12. Mullen HS, Scavelli TD, Quesenberry KE, et al. Gastrointestinal foreign body in ferrets: 25 cases (1986–1990). J Am Anim Hosp Assoc 1989;28:13–9.
13. Burgess M, Garner M. Clinical aspects of inflammatory bowel disease in ferrets. Exotic DVM 2002;4(2):29–34.
14. Hoppes S, Xenoulis PG, Berghoff N, et al. Serum cobalamin, folate, and methylmalonic acid concentrations in ferrets *(Mustela putorius)*. In: Proceedings of Assoc of Exotic Mammal Veterinarians 2008.
15. Quesenberry KE, Rosenthal KL. Ferrets: endocrine diseases. In: Quesenberry KE, Carpenter JW, editors. Ferrets, rabbits and rodents: clinical medicine and surgery. 2nd edition. Philadelphia: WD Saunders; 2003. p. 79–90.
16. Shoemaker NJ, Schuurmans M, Moorman H. Correlation between age at neutering and at onset of hyperadrenocorticism in ferrets. J Am Vet Med Assoc 2000; 216(2):195–7.
17. Rosenthal KL, Peterson ME, Quesenberry KE, et al. Hyperadrenocorticism associated with adrenocortical tumor or nodular hyperplasia of the adrenal gland in ferrets: 50 cases (1987–1991). J Am Vet Med Assoc 1993;203(2):271–5.
18. Antinoff N, Hahn K. Ferret oncology: diseases, diagnostics and therapeutics. Vet Clin North Am Exotic Anim Pract 2004;7:579–625.
19. Rosenthal KL, Peterson ME. Plasma androgen concentrations in ferrets with adrenal gland disease. J Am Vet Med Assoc 1996;209:1097–102.
20. Wagner RA, Bailey EM, Schneider JF, et al. Leuprolide acetate treatment of adrenocortical disease in ferrets. J Am Vet Med Assoc 2001;218:1272–4.
21. Ramer JC, Benson KG, Morrisey JK, et al. Effects of melatonin administration on the clinical course of adrenocortical disease in domestic ferrets. J Am Vet Med Assoc 2006;229(11):1743–8.
22. Weiss C. Medical management of ferret adrenal tumors and hyperplasia. Exotic DVM 1999;1(5):38–9.
23. Li X, Fox JG, Padrid PA. Neoplastic disease in ferrets: 574 cases (1968–1997). J Am Vet Med Assoc 1998;212(1):1402–6.
24. Li X, Fox JG. Neoplastic diseases. In: Fox JG, editor. Biology and diseases of the ferret. Baltimore (MD): Williams & Wilkins; 1998. p. 405–47.
25. Weiss CA, Williams BH, Scott MV. Insulinoma in the ferret: clinical findings and treatment comparison of 66 cases. J Am Anim Hosp Assoc 1998;34(6):471–5.

26. Caplan ER, Peterson ME, Mullen HS, et al. Diagnosis and treatment of insulin-secreting pancreatic islet cell tumors in ferrets: 57 cases (1986–1994). J Am Vet Med Assoc 1996;209(10):1741–5.
27. Erdman SE, Kanki PJ, Moore FM, et al. Clusters of lymphoma in ferrets. Cancer Invest 1996;14(3):225–30.
28. Erdman SE, Reimann KA, Moore FM, et al. Transmission of a chronic lymphopro-liferative syndrome in ferrets. Lab Invest 1995;72(5):539–46.
29. Williams BH, Weiss CA. Ferrets: neoplasia. In: Quesenberry KE, Carpenter JW, editors. Ferrets, rabbits and rodents: clinical medicine and surgery. 2nd edition. Philadelphia: WD Saunders; 2003. p. 91–106.
30. Erdman SE, Brown SA, Kawasaki TA, et al. Clinical and pathologic findings in ferrets with lymphoma: 60 cases (1982–1994). J Am Vet Med Assoc 1996; 108(8):1285–9.
31. Petrie JP, Morrisey JK. Ferrets: cardiovascular and other diseases. In: Quesenberry KE, Carpenter JW, editors. Ferrets, rabbits and rodents: clinical medicine and surgery. 2nd edition. Philadelphia: WD Saunders; 2003. p. 58–71.
32. Fox JG. Other systemic diseases. In: Fox JG, editor. Biology and diseases of the ferret. Baltimore (MD): Williams & Wilkins; 1998. p. 313–20.
33. Wagner R. Ferret cardiology. Vet Clin North Am Exot Anim Pract 2009;12:115–34.
34. Antinoff N. Clinical observations in ferrets with naturally occurring heartworm disease and preliminary evaluation of treatment with ivermectin with and without Melarsomine. Recent Adv Heartworm Dis; 2002. p. 45–7.
35. Kawasaki TA. Normal parameters and laboratory interpretation of disease states in the domestic ferret. Semin Avian Exotic Pet Med 1994;3(1):40–7.
36. Fisher PG. Exotic mammal renal disease: causes and clinical presentation. Vet Clin North Am Exotic Anim Pract 2006;9:33–43.
37. Orcutt CJ. Ferret urogenital diseases. Vet Clin North Am Exot Anim Pract 2003; 6(1):113–38.
38. Polluck CG. Ferrets: urogenital diseases. In: Quesenberry KE, Carpenter JW, editors. Ferrets, rabbits and rodents: clinical medicine and surgery. 2nd edition. Philadelphia: WD Saunders; 2003. p. 41–9.
39. Williams BH. Pathology of the domestic ferret (Mustela putorius furo). In: 2004 C.L. Davis ACVP Symposium Pathology of Non-traditional Pets; 2004. p. 103–32.
40. Fox JA, Parson RC, Bell JA. Diseases of the genitourinary system. In: Fox JG, editor. Biology and diseases of the ferret. Baltimore (MD): Williams & Wilkins; 1998. p. 247–72.
41. Cathers TE, Isaza R, Oehme F. Acute ibuprofen toxicosis in a ferret. J Am Vet Med Assoc 2000;216(9):1426–8.
42. Richardson JA, Balabuszko RA. Ibuprofen ingestion in a ferret. Exotic DVM 2001; 3(2):3.
43. Richardson JA, Balabuszko RA. Managing ferret toxicosis. Exotic DVM 2000;2(4): 23–6.
44. Straube EF, Schuster NH, Sinclair AJ. Zinc toxicity in the ferret. J Comp Pathol 1980;90(3):355–61.
45. Fox JG, Zeman DH, Mortimer JD, et al. Copper toxicosis in sibling ferrets. J Am Vet Med Assoc 1994;205(8):1154–6.
46. Van der Woerdt A. Ophthalmologic diseases in small pet mammals. In: Quesenberry KE, Carpenter JW, editors. Ferrets, rabbits and rodents: clinical medicine and surgery. 2nd edition. Philadelphia: WD Saunders; 2003. p. 421–7.
47. Erdman SE, Xiantang L, Fox JG. Hematopoietic diseases. In: Fox JG, editor. Biology and diseases of the ferret. Baltimore (MD): Williams & Wilkins; 1998. p. 231–46.

Care of the Geriatric Rabbit

Angela M. Lennox, DVM, Dipl. ABVP-Avian

KEYWORDS

• Rabbit • Geriatric • Arthritis • Dental disease

Exotic companion mammal veterinarians are seeing an extension of life spans of pet rabbits seen in practice. The average life span reported in laboratory and lay literature for the domestic rabbit is 5 to 10 years. The author and others are now regularly seeing rabbits living to 9 or 10 years, the oldest reported in the author's practice being 14 years.

Rabbits are herbivorous prey species with continually growing (elodont) teeth.[1] This feature allows the geriatric rabbit to possess teeth that are essentially "new," a distinct advantage over geriatric carnivores. In the wild, longevity is not naturally achieved by prey species. Expanded longevity is generally desirable; however, it necessarily accompanies an increase in geriatric disorders. An improved understanding of geriatric disorders in pet rabbits allows early recognition and the opportunity to improve quality of life.

WELL CARE FOR GERIATRIC RABBITS

Opinions vary as to recommended frequency of examinations for apparently well older rabbits. The author prefers to begin biannual examinations with analysis of the complete blood count and biochemistry panel at age 5 years, with examinations increasing as age and condition indicate. The stress of presentation for examination and phlebotomy should be weighed against the advantage of frequent evaluation.

CHRONIC RENAL FAILURE

Chronic renal failure is common in rabbits, and is often recognized during an episode of acute failure.[2] Whereas acute renal failure (sudden onset of filtration failure characterized by accumulation of uremic toxins and fluid/electrolyte and acid/base imbalance) can be characterized as pre-, post-, and intrinsic renal, most acute failures in older rabbits are an acute episode of a chronic intrinsic renal failure.[2] Clinical signs and symptoms may be subtle, but may include dehydration, polyuria/polydypsia, weight loss, failure to groom, anorexia, and depression. There are numerous causes of chronic renal disease in rabbits, but some are primarily identified only in laboratory

Avian and Exotic Animal Clinic, 9330 Waldemar Road, Indianapolis, IN 46268, USA
E-mail address: birddr@aol.com

Vet Clin Exot Anim 13 (2010) 123–133
doi:10.1016/j.cvex.2009.09.002
1094-9194/10/$ – see front matter © 2010 Elsevier Inc. All rights reserved.

animals, for example, feeding of diets with excessive vitamin D and calcium. Other causes include urolithiasis, bacterial infections, neoplasia, and nephrocalcinosis.[2]

Encephalitozoon cuniculi (ECUN) has been demonstrated to produce mild to severe interstitial nephritis. A recent study of histopathologic examinations of pet rabbits that died or were euthanized showed that of 48 rabbits with ECUN spores detected in the brain, 39 also had interstitial nephritis; 89.6% of renal lesions were described as chronic, whereas the rest were acute. However, the same study showed that the degree of severity of lesions did not always correlate with the degree of clinical symptoms.[3] Antemortem diagnosis of ECUN as a cause of renal failure in rabbits is difficult, but can be supported with serology and protein electrophoresis.[4]

Management of acute renal failure is similar to that for other species.[5] Management of chronic renal failure is supportive. Some cases benefit from long-term administration of subcutaneous fluids and hand feeding. The GIF Tube Implant kit is a silicone catheter designed for long-term implantation in the subcutis for administration of fluids (GIF-Tube, PractiVet, Phoenix, AZ). Though designed for dogs and cats, the author and others have used this product in rabbits with chronic renal failure requiring longer-term at-home subcutaneous administration of fluid (see Hospice and end-of-life issues later in this article) (**Fig. 1**). The manufacturer provides a demonstration CD of implantation instructions for practitioners and at-home use for owners.

Erythropoietin has been administered to rabbits with secondary anemia.[2]

The author has encountered numerous rabbits experiencing good quality of life for many months, despite muscle wasting and persistently elevated blood urea nitrogen and creatinine.

CARDIOVASCULAR DISEASE

Cardiovascular disease is gaining recognition in exotic companion mammals as the level of veterinary care increases and patients age. The rabbit is a model for atherosclerosis in humans, as lesions are readily produced by feeding a diet high in fat.[6] However, little is known about naturally occurring disease in the pet rabbit.

The thoracic cavity and lungs of the rabbit are exceptionally small in comparison with those of other similar-sized animals. Severe reduction in pulmonary mass (as in mediastinal tumors) does not seem to produce symptoms until late in the course of the disease. Therefore, it is likely the rabbit may not exhibit cardiac-related respiratory symptoms until late in the course of the disease. Symptoms can include depression, exercise intolerance, and increased respiratory rate and effort, which in the author's experience may be absent at rest and significantly worse with exercise.

Diagnosis of heart disease is enhanced with radiography and cardiac ultrasonography, which is important to better characterize heart disease and determine treatment options. Normal parameters for echocardiography have been described.[7]

Cardiac conditions reported in the rabbit include valvular disease (endocardiosis) and cardiomyopathy. Several diseases have been reported to cause cardiomyopathy in the laboratory rabbit, but incidence in pet rabbits is unknown, and likely to be low.

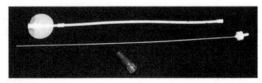

Fig. 1. The GIF Tube Implant kit.

These include nutritional deficiencies (vitamin E deficiency), viral (coronavirus), bacterial (salmonellosis or pasteurellosis), or protozoal (ECUN) infections, and toxins.[7,8]

Excessive stress may produce heart disease. Stress causes catecholamine release in rabbits, and when sustained can result in coronary vessel constriction with ischemic cardiomyopathy.[7]

Treatment of congestive heart failure relies on use of drugs traditionally used in canine medicine, and are based on anecdotal reports of success.[2] Drugs used by the author for management of cardiac disease are listed in **Table 1**. Drug dosages should be adapted to clinical response and improvement of echocardiographic results. The use of taurine has been shown to improve cardiovascular function in laboratory rabbits with induced cardiac failure (see **Table 1**).

Vascular disease can produce hypertension. Indirect blood pressure is determined using an ultrasonic Doppler and pediatric cuff (width 30%–40% of the diameter of the limb circumference) usually placed proximal to the carpus. Acquiring an audible pulse with the Doppler requires significant practice; initial difficulty encountered should not discourage the practitioner from developing this skill. The author and others normally note blood pressures in normal patients between 110 and 180 mm Hg using this method.

ARTHRITIS/DEGENERATIVE JOINT DISEASE

Osteoarthritis and vertebral spondylosis are commonly encountered in older rabbits. Associated signs and symptoms include reluctance to move, urine/fecal staining due to inability to clean and properly direct the urine stream, and lameness.

The rabbit is a laboratory model for trauma-induced arthritis and response to drug therapy. In rabbits whose legs were immobilized with plaster casts, those receiving intra-articular injections of 0.3 mL hyaluronic acid showed significant reduction of cartilage degeneration when compared with rabbits receiving a saline injection.[9] Similar effects (retardation of progression of osteoarthritis) were seen in rabbits undergoing anterior cruciate ligament transection that were injected with an intra-articular mixture of glucose or dextrose, amino acids, and ascorbic acid 5 times weekly.[10]

Table 1 Drug dosages for geriatric rabbits		
Drug	**Dosage (mg/kg)**	**Comments**
Meloxicam[28]	0.2–0.3 IM, PO SID	Some report higher dosages required for more chronic pain; monitor renal values throughout treatment[21]
Ketoprofen[28]	3 every 24 h IM	
Carprofen[28]	4–5 every 24 h PO	
Furosemide[29]	1–4 every 4–6 h IM	
Enalapril[7]	0.5 every 12–24 h PO	
Digoxin[29]	0.005–0.01 every 24–48 h PO	
Pimobendam[7]	0.1–0.3 every 12–24 h PO	
Taurine[30]	100 SID PO	Has demonstrated improvement in cardiac function in rabbits with artificially induced heart failure

Consider dose reduction in rabbits with renal and/or hepatic disease.
Abbreviations: BSAVA, British Small Animal Veterinary Association; IM, intramuscular; PO, by mouth; SID, once a day.

Other drugs shown to reduce degenerative changes in rabbit osteoarthritis models include intra-articular administered sodium hyaluronate and orally administered glucosamine hydrochloride, 100 mg by mouth daily.[11–13]

Several studies exist on the use of joint health products in dogs, and include glucosamine, chondroitin, P54FP (Indian and Javanese tumeric extract), green-lipped mussels, and ω-3 fatty acids.[14] Results are variable; however, a systematic review of the literature showed that there is moderate evidence that some joint health products (JHPs), including green-lipped mussels products, P54FP, a combination of chondroitin sulfate, glucosamine hydrochloride, and manganese ascorbate, provide some benefit.[14] The author is unaware of studies on the effects of JHPs in rabbits with naturally occurring disease.

Product recommendation can be difficult, and dosing is extrapolated from other species. The ACCLAIM system has been proposed as a means for veterinarians to evaluate the label claims and quality of specific JHPs (**Table 2**).[15]

Housing should be optimized for rabbits with spondylosis or joint disease. Nonslip, soft surfaces are beneficial, as the force produced by hopping is much higher than that produced by walking. Lowering one side of the litter box allows easier access. Owners must be instructed to clean the perineum daily (see later discussion on perineal dermatitis).

Table 2		
ACCLAIM system for rapid evaluation of joint health product labels[15]		
A	A name you recognize?	Products manufactured by an established company that provides educational materials for veterinarians or other consumers are prerable to joint health products manufactured by a new company
C	Clinical experience	Companies that support clinical research and have their products used in clinical trials that are published in peer-reviewed journals to which veterinarians have access are more likely to have a quality product
C	Contents	All ingredients should be clearly indicated on the label
L	Label claims	Label claims that sound too good to be true probably are. Products with realistic label claims based on results of scientific studies, rather than testimonials, are more likely to be reputable. Products with illegal claims (claim to diagnose, treat, cure, or prevent a disease) should be avoided
A	Administration recommendations	Dosing instructions should be accurate and easy to follow; it should be easy to calculate the amount of active ingredient administered per dose per day
I	Identification of lot	A lot identification number or some other tracking system indicates that a premarket or postmarket surveillance system exits to ensure product quality. In addition, companies that have voluntarily instituted current good manufacturing practices and other quality-control or quality-assurance techniques (eg, tamper-resistant packaging of identification of individual tablets or capsules) provide evidence of long-term investment in the product and company
M	Manufacturer information	Basic company information should be clearly stated on the label. Preferably, this should include a Web site or details for contacting customer support

From Oke S. Oral joint supplements. The Horse 2008; May 1; with permission.

DENTAL DISEASE

Dental disease is not necessarily associated with aging in rabbits. Many older rabbits manage to avoid acquired dental disease and possess essentially normal, continually renewing teeth well into old age. Other older rabbits may develop varying patterns of dental disease apparently related to slowing or cessation of tooth growth, which may be due to attrition of the alveolus. Severe acquired dental disease, however, is primarily a disease of younger rabbits; in these patients, evidence of dental disease is often apparent before 3 years of age.[1] Accurate diagnosis and excellent owner compliance can result in adequate disease management and acquisition of normal expected life span; in many cases these patients eventually die of diseases unrelated to those of dentition. The author and others frequently see geriatric rabbits that have had years of regular dental care. In some cases all teeth are eventually lost, and patients survive with good to excellent quality of life on a diet of liquid Critical Care (Oxbow Animal Health, Murdoch, NE). Diagnosis and treatment of dental disease is presented in great detail elsewhere.[1]

SPLAY LEG

Several practitioners have reported unilateral or bilateral abduction of the thoracic limbs in older, often larger breed rabbits (**Fig. 2**). The condition seems to be associated with muscle wasting and is generally progressive. Housing on nonslick surfaces is helpful.

MUSCLE WASTING

Though not a primary disease disorder, muscle wasting and moderate to severe weight loss is a common feature in aged rabbits. Causes are varied, and can include chronic renal failure and acquired dental disease. A thorough approach is required to discover the underlying etiology.

Supplemental feeding is often beneficial. Critical Care can be offered in a dish or via syringe feeding. The manufacturer provides detailed instructions for product use.

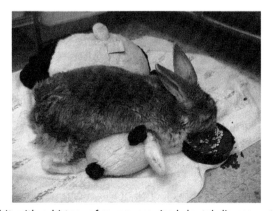

Fig. 2. Older rabbit with a history of severe acquired dental disease, retrobulbar abscess, and enucleation of the right eye. The rabbit survived with good quality of life for several years on Oxbow Critical Care and soaked pellets. Worsening splay leg of the thoracic limbs resulted in decreased mobility. The owner used towels and a stuffed animal to support the pet during brief hospice care at home before ultimately choosing euthanasia.

OCULAR LESIONS

Age-related ocular lesions, including cataract formation, are common in rabbits. Current literature suggests a high percentage of ocular lesions may be caused by ECUN.

A 2005 study describing histologic features of ECUN-induced ocular lesions in rabbits demonstrated intraocular locally extensive pyogranulomatous infiltration of the posterior chamber with disruption of the anterior lens capsule. Spores were identified via immunohistochemical staining in all cases.[16] Another study described ocular lesions as phacoclastic uveitis. All samples from abnormal eyes (n = 10) obtained via enucleation or phacoemulsification were positive for ECUN via the polymerase chain reaction.[17]

CHRONIC OTITIS

Stenosis of the ear canal is a common finding in aged lop-eared rabbits. In the author's experience, all older lop-eared rabbits have some degree of stenosis, which predisposes to otitis. Disease is difficult to manage medically due to abnormal anatomy. Lateral ear canal resection, ostectomy, and total ear canal ablation may be required in selected cases.[18]

ULCERATIVE PODODERMATITIS AND PERINEAL DERMATITIS

Pododermatitis can be encountered in rabbits of any age, and is often a result of improper husbandry (wire-bottom cages, inadequate cleaning); however, any condition impairing ability to groom normally and exposure to urine/feces due to decreased mobility can contribute. Inability to groom also leads to perineal accumulation of feces and urine and dermatitis, or scalding.

It is important to address the underlying cause of decreased mobility. Pododermatitis is treated with local wound management (debridement, flushing with or without bandaging), housing on soft surfaces, and antibiotics plus analgesics. Underlying immunocompromise and wasting can delay or prevent healing in some cases. Severe cases with pus and involvement of tendons, ligaments, and joints may require surgical intervention, including amputation, which should be considered carefully in the geriatric rabbit.

Perineal dermatitis is treated the same as any other infected wound, with careful clipping of the hair, cleansing and application of antibiotics, and use of soothing ointments or products designed to promote healing once infection has resolved and granulation has begun. Some elderly rabbits benefit from regular preventative shaving of the perineum in order to allow the owner to cleanse more effectively. The author prefers dilute chlorhexidine and application of silver sulfadiazine cream (SSD, Par Pharmaceutical, Shreveport, LA), Zinc products (Zn7 Derm, Addison Biological Laboratory Inc, Fayette, MO), or healing products (Heal-X Soother Plus Cream or Spray, Zoological Education Network, Lake Worth, FL).

NEOPLASIA

Neoplasia occurs in rabbits, and incidence of all neoplasms increases with age. The most commonly encountered neoplasm is uterine adenocarcinoma. Uterine adenocarcinoma can produce few signs until the disease is advanced. The most commonly reported sign is hematuria, and uterine masses are often palpable. The abnormal uterus may be palpable, and metastasis, especially to liver and lungs, can occur in some cases.[19]

The most common clinical presentation of thymoma is bilateral exophthalmos, which may worsen with exercise or excitation. Respiratory symptoms usually occur later in the course of the disease. Treatment options include surgery and radiation.[20]

MODIFICATION OF THERAPEUTICS IN GERIATRIC RABBITS

In human medicine, drug dosages are often adjusted for geriatric patients due to assumed decrease in renal and hepatic function.[21] Although specific recommendations for geriatric rabbits are unavailable, drug dosage modification should be considered, especially when organ disease has been positively identified.

Chronic renal failure impacts drug metabolism; therefore, adjustments in drug dosages should be considered in patients with chronic renal failure. In humans, various strategies for estimation of glomerular filtration rate (GFR) are used for "adjusting the dosage of medications excreted by glomerular filtration."[21] For example, in human patients with impaired clearance, dosage of butorphanol is adjusted to half the normal dose. Although estimation of GFR is unavailable for rabbit patients, serious consideration should be given to lowering dosages of all drugs, in particular, any drugs metabolized by glomerular filtration in rabbits with suspected renal insufficiency. Drugs more commonly used in rabbits metabolized at least partially via glomerular filtration include sulfonamides such as trimethoprim sulfamethoxazole.

While procaine penicillin is excreted via tubular secretion, impaired renal function causes delayed excretion in humans and other species. Meloxicam is metabolized by the liver. Use is not recommended in humans and tested animal patients that are dehydrated, or have liver or renal disease (due to reduction of blood flow to the kidneys).[22]

SEDATION AND ANESTHESIA FOR THE GERIATRIC RABBIT

Human anesthesiologists routinely modify protocols and drug dosages for the elderly. A geriatric rabbit otherwise in good health may not necessarily represent a serious anesthetic risk; however, clinicians must assume some alteration of cardiovascular and renal health with advancing age.

Certain drugs should be avoided in older patients. Medetomidine (Pfizer Animal Health, New York, NY) is listed frequently as a choice for pre-anesthesia and anesthesia in the rabbit.[23] A few studies have demonstrated use in rabbits, but use in elderly patients has not been investigated. It should be noted that medetomidine and dexmedetomidine are contraindicated in dogs or cats with cardiovascular disease, respiratory disease, liver or kidney disease, or in any debilitated patient.[24] Therefore, use in the geriatric rabbit should be avoided or used cautiously.

The author and others prefer a balanced approach to sedation and anesthesia for all exotic animal patients, including pre-anesthesia, analgesia, local/regional analgesia, and anesthesia if required. Use of a balanced approach allows for reduction of any single agent, including inhalant agents, thus increasing patient safety. Many brief procedures producing minimal discomfort can be accomplished with sedation only, for example, radiography, placement of an intravenous catheter, and clipping or minor wound care.[25] In geriatric patients, dosages of all drugs are reduced depending on patient condition.

For geriatric patients in which the need for sedation/anesthesia for diagnostic or therapeutic procedures outweigh the risks, the author has had great success with the combination of midazolam with an opioid (butorphanol, buprenorphine, hydromorphone, fentanyl), with the addition of low-dose ketamine if required (**Table 3**). The addition of local analgesia with lidocaine, 1 mg/kg as a local or regional block is

Table 3
Anesthetic and analgesic drugs used by the author in geriatric rabbits

Drug	Dosage (mg/kg)	Comments
Midazolam	0.25 IM	
Butorphanol	0.10–0.20 IM	
Buprenorphine	0.04 IM	
Hydromorphone	0.10 IM	
Ketamine	1–10 IM	
Etomidate	1–2 IV	Must be combined with benzodiazepine to prevent muscle tremors

Consider further dose reduction in rabbits with renal and/or hepatic disease.
Abbreviations: IM, intramuscular; IV, intravenous.

extremely beneficial. When additional anesthesia is required, inhalant isoflurane or sevoflurane can be added at minimal effective concentrations.

An alternative is the use of injectable etomidate combined with midazolam. Etomidate is commonly used in geriatric and high-risk human patients, and is apparently unaffected by impaired renal function.[26] Etomidate must be injected intravenously, and combined with a benzodiazepine to prevent temporary tetany and seizures. Onset of action is immediate, and duration is approximately 5 to 7 minutes in rabbits and other mammals. The author's experience with this drug has been overwhelmingly positive, even in patients with advanced disease conditions. However, death occurred in a single geriatric rabbit with suspected advanced cardiac disease.

HOSPICE AND END-OF-LIFE ISSUES

Significant attention has been directed toward hospice, or palliative end-of-life care for companion animals. A recent Internet search revealed numerous businesses offering hospice services for traditional pets. The concept of hospice care can be applied to aged rabbits as well.

In general, the hospice setting should be clean, quiet, and stress-free. If possible, ill or dying rabbits should not be separated from bonded companions, and the author is unaware of situations in which bullying or harassment has occurred. Bedding should provide traction, be soft, absorbent, and easy to clean. Hospital absorbent pads are ideal (Wings Maxima Disposable Underpads, Tyco Healthcare) (**Fig. 3**). Food and water bowls and bottles are placed within easy reach. Caloric and fluid needs can be supplied through syringe feeding of Critical Care formula as per manufacturer's instructions. Nasogastric tube feeding can be considered for those rabbits unable or unwilling to eat; however, stress associated with this procedure should strongly be considered. Nasogastric feeding should be considered a temporary measure only.

Some rabbits benefit from administration of fluids, either subcutaneously or intravenously. Willing owners can be instructed to do either in the home setting. In selected cases, an implanted subcutaneous catheter is beneficial (see earlier section on Chronic renal failure).

Daily care also includes gentle cleaning of the perineum to prevent scalding. In rabbits with chronic epiphora, accumulations of secretions should be removed frequently to avoid dermatitis. Rabbits unwilling or unable to groom may benefit from shaving of the hair of the perineum in order to reduce fecal and urine accumulation and allow owners to more effectively cleanse the area.

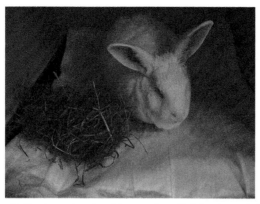

Fig. 3. Ill rabbit hospitalized on absorbent human hospital "underpads." Pads help prevent urine accumulation and scalding.

Analgesia for hospice patients should emphasize optimal pain control, with lesser regard for untoward systemic effects.

TECHNIQUES FOR EUTHANASIA

Choosing the time for euthanasia is difficult in most circumstances, and is particularly complicated in rabbits due to their inherent tendency to hide signs of illness. A significant change in routine, and unwillingness to eat or accept treats or groom are clear indications of distress in rabbits. In situations whereby their condition is unlikely to improve, euthanasia should be considered.

Humane, stress-free euthanasia requires careful planning and implementation, especially when the owners wish to be present. The American Veterinary Medical Association Guidelines on Euthanasia for rabbits suggest the following: barbiturates, CO_2, CO, or potassium chloride in conjunction with general anesthesia. Other listed acceptable techniques such as cervical dislocation are unacceptable to most veterinary staff and owners.[27] The author prefers the following technique, especially when owners wish to be present: induction with medetomidine at 50 µg/kg, and ketamine, 30 mg/kg administered intramuscularly. Owners are encouraged to hold their pet

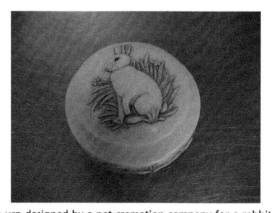

Fig. 4. Decorative urn designed by a pet cremation company for a rabbit.

during induction as comfort level allows. Smaller doses may be repeated if necessary. Once deep anesthesia is achieved with no response to toe pinch, euthanasia solution is administered intravenously or by cardiac puncture.

Owners should be given options regarding disposition of the pet after euthanasia. Frequently chosen options include home burial (local ordinances permitting), and private or group cremation. Most small animal cremation companies are willing to provide services to owners of rabbits and other exotic pets (**Fig. 4**).

REFERENCES

1. Capello V, Gracis M. In: Lennox AM, editor. Rabbit and rodent dentistry. Hoboken (NJ): Wiley-Blackwell (Formerly Zoologic Education Network); 2005.
2. Pare JA, Paul-Murphy J. Disorders of the reproductive and urinary systems, in Quesenbery KE, Carpenter JW, editors. Ferrets, rabbits and rodents, clinical medicine and surgery. St. Louis (MO): Saunders; 2004. p. 183–93.
3. Csokai J, Grube A, Kunzel F, et al. Encephalitozoonosis in pet rabbits (*Oryctolagus cuniculus*): pathohistological findings in animals with latent infection versus clinical manifestation. Parasitol Res 2009;104(3):629–35.
4. Cray C, Arcia G, Kelleher S, et al. Application of ELISA and protein electrophoresis in the diagnosis of *Encephalitozoon cuniculi* infection in rabbits. Am J Vet Res 2009;70(4):478–82.
5. Paul-Murphy J. Critical care of the rabbit. Vet Clin Exot Anim 2007;10:437–61.
6. Finking G, Hanke H. Nikolaj Nikolajewitsch Antischkow established the cholesterol-fed rabbit as a model for atherosclerosis research. Atherosclerosis 1997;135:1–7.
7. Pariaut R. Cardiovascular physiology and diseases of the rabbit. Vet Clin Exotic Anim 2009;12:135–44.
8. Harcourt-Brown F. Cardiorespiratory disease. In: Textbook of rabbit medicine. London: Elsevier Science Limited; 2002. p. 324–34.
9. Liang MH, Shang H, Sun L, et al. Preventive effect of hyaluronic acid on degerative articular cartilage of immobilized rabbit knees. J Clin Rehab Tissue Engineering Research 2007;11(45):9043–6.
10. Park YS, Lim SW, Lee IH, et al. Intra-articular injection of a nutritive mixture solution protects articular cartilage from osteoarthritic progression induced by anterior cruciate ligament transection in mature rabbits: a randomized controlled trial. Arthritis Research Therapy 2007;9:R8.
11. Zhang SZ, Wu YH. The effect of sodium hyaluronate on the rabbit osteoarthrosis. Shanghai Kou Qiang Yi Xue 2003;12(3):187–90.
12. Wang SX, Laverty S, Dumitriu M, et al. The effects of glucosamine hydrochloride on subchondral bone changes in an animal model of osteoarthritis. Arthritis Rheum 2007;56(5):1527–48.
13. Harcourt-Brown F. Skin diseases. In: Textbook of rabbit medicine. London: Elsevier Science Limited; 2002. p. 224–48.
14. Aragon CL, Hofmeister EH, Budsberg SC. Systematic review of clinical trials of treatments for osteoarthritis in dogs. J AmVet Med Assoc 2007;250:514–21.
15. Oke S. Indications and contraindications for the use of orally administered joint health products in dogs and cats. J Am Vet Med Assoc 2009;234(11):1393–7.
16. Giordano C, Weigt A, Vercelli A, et al. Immunohistochemical identification of *Encephalitozoon cuniculi* in phacoclastic uveitis in four rabbits. Vet Opthal 2005; 8(4):271–5.
17. Csokai J, Joachim A, Gruber A, et al. Diagnostic markers for encephalitozoonosis in pet rabbits. Vet Parsitol 2009;163(1–2):18–26.

18. Capello V. Surgical treatment of otitis externa and media in pet rabbits. ExoticDVM 2004;6(3):15–21.

19. Harcourt-Brown F. Urinogenital diseases. In: Textbook of rabbit medicine. London: Elsevier Science Limited; 2002. p. 335–51.

20. Sanchez-Migallon DG, Mayer J, Gould J, et al. Radiation therapy for the treatment of thymoma in rabbits. J Exotic pet Med 2006;15(2):138–44.

21. Spruill WJ, Wade WE, Cobbii HH. Estimating glomerular filtration rate with a new equation:application to pharmacy and drug dosing. Am J Health Syst Pharm 2007;64(9):916.

22. Turner PV, Chen HC, Taylor WM. Pharmacokinetis of meloxicam in rabbits after single and repeat oral dosing. Comp Med 2006;56(1):63–7.

23. Grint NJ, Murison PJ. A comparison of ketamine-midazolam and ketamine-medetomidine combinations for induction of anesthesia in rabbits. Vet Anaesth Analg 2008;35(2):113–21.

24. Dexdomitor veterinary product information. Available at: www.drugs.com/vet/dexdomitor.html. Accessed May 5, 2009.

25. Lennox AM. It's great to sedate. Proceedings North Am Vet Conference, Orlando FL, 2009.

26. Etomidate Veterinary Product Information. Available at: www.drugs.com/vet/etomidate.html. Accessed June, 2009.

27. AVMA guidelines on euthanasia. 2007 American Veterinary Medical Association. Available at: www.avma.org/issues/animal_welfare/euthanasia.pdf. Accessed May 13, 2009.

28. Meredith A, Crossley DA. Rabbits. In: Meredith A, Redrobe S, editors. BSAVA manual of exotic pets. 4th edition. Gloucester (UK): British Small Animal Medical Association; 2002. p. 76–92.

29. Carpenter JW. Rabbits. In: Exotic animal formulary. St. Louis (MO): Elsevier; 2005. p. 411–42.

30. Takihaa K, Azuma J, Awata N, et al. Beneficial effect of taurine in rabbits with chronic congestive heart failure. Am Heart J 1986;112(6):1278–84.

Pathology of Aging Psittacines

Drury R. Reavill, DVM, DABVP-Avian, DACVP[a],*,
Gerry M. Dorrestein, DVM, PhD, DVP[b]

KEYWORDS

- Psittacines • Geriatric • Atherosclerosis • Lung fibrosis
- Neoplasia • Cataract • Chronic liver disease

Aging is the accumulation of progressive cellular changes typically associated with decreased physiologic function. These changes result in generalized impairment of physiologic functions, a decreased ability to respond to stresses, an increased risk of age-associated disease, and an increased likelihood of death. This phenomenon is universal to all living things, although life span and life expectancy differ among species and even among individual members of a species.

Birds are prone to many of the same diseases that afflict aging mammals, including waning fertility, cardiovascular disease, cancers, cataracts, and osteoarthritis. Although few studies or reviews have examined the process of aging in our personable and relatively long-lived parrots, generally they appear to have aging rates that are much slower than those for similar-sized mammals.[1–4]

PHYSIOLOGY

Surprisingly, birds, bats, and a few other organisms with high metabolic rates have some of the slowest rates of senescence.[5] In general, birds live long and age slowly, despite their high metabolic rates (1.5–2.5 times higher than similar-sized mammals) and very high total lifetime energy expenditures, which may be five or more times higher that those of mammals.[1,6–8]

Birds seem to have evolved specific adaptations for combating oxidative and glycoxydative processes thought to be the primary causes of aging-related cellular damage.[1,9–16]

Current theories of senescence suggest that wear and tear at the cellular level (oxidative and glycoxydative stress and telomere shortening or other genetic damage) result in damage that cannot be repaired.[17–21] An extended life span is expected in individuals with large amounts of antioxidants, as such antioxidants prevent free

[a] Zoo/Exotic Pathology Service, 7647 Wachtel Way, Citrus Heights, CA 95610, USA
[b] Diagnostic Pathology Laboratorium NOIVBD, Wintelresedijk 51, NL-5507 PP Veldhoven, The Netherlands
* Corresponding author.
E-mail address: Dreavill@zooexotic.com (D.R. Reavill).

Vet Clin Exot Anim 13 (2010) 135–150
doi:10.1016/j.cvex.2009.12.001
1094-9194/10/$ – see front matter © 2010 Elsevier Inc. All rights reserved.

radical–induced cell injury and facilitate repair.[5,22,23] The effect of telomere length is less well associated with cellular senescence. Telomeres are conserved nucleotide sequences essential for replication by ensuring complete replication of chromosomal ends and protecting the chromosomal termini from fusion and degradation. Chromosomal telomeres have been shown to shorten with age in somatic cells of humans, and are implicated in cellular senescence in mice.[24–26] One study has found avian telomeric DNA sequences (from 18 species and subspecies of birds in several different orders) to be five- to 10-fold longer than in mammals.[27] Two studies found telomere length was not reliably correlated with aging rates or life spans in birds.[24,28] However, other works have reported a positive correlation between age-related changes in telomere lengths in several bird species with markedly different life spans.[29–31]

OVERVIEW

This article includes a summary of disease conditions in older psittacines submitted to a private exotic species pathology service, Zoo/Exotic Pathology Service (ZEPS) in West Sacramento, California (**Table 1**). This is not meant to represent a true prevalence of the disease in this population, as there will be a bias due to decisions (perceived value of the information to the practitioner or client) in submitting cases for pathologic examination. The population chosen includes commonly kept species having adequate numbers of submissions. Small birds, such as budgerigars (*Melopsittacus undulatus*) and lovebirds (*Agapornis* sp) were considered elderly at 6 years; cockatiels (*Nymphycus hollandicus*) at 12 years; and large psittacines, such as Amazon parrots (*Amazona* sp), macaws (*Ara* sp), cockatoos (*Cacatua* sp), and African grey parrots (*Psittacus erithacus*), at 30 years. These are somewhat arbitrary assignments but based on life-span reports in the literature.[32,33] Lesions were tabulated. However, not all submissions had a complete set of tissues to examine and many birds had multiple lesions considered to be age-related. In summary, some of the typical changes seen in aging mammals (eg, chronic interstitial nephritis) are not so often seen in birds (**Fig. 1**). However, some disease problems are seen more often in older birds than in younger ones.

DISEASES BY ORGAN SYSTEM
Cardiovascular Disease

A number of aging changes to the heart are well recognized in mammals, especially humans. These include increasing epicardial fat, hypertrophic changes to the left ventricle associated with hypertension, calcification of the valves, a loss of myocytes, an increase in collagenized connective tissue, and the accumulation of intracytoplasmic lipofuscin. Cardiac disease has been historically underdiagnosed in pet birds. However, with increasing use of radiography, electrocardiography, and echocardiography, cardiac disease has been found to occur more often than previously assumed.[34]

The two disease conditions best described in the aging psittacine heart include atherosclerosis and lipofuscin accumulation.

Atherosclerosis

Atherosclerosis is reported most often in Amazon parrots, particularly the blue-fronted Amazon parrot (*Amazona aestiva aestiva*); African grey parrots; and macaws. Atherosclerosis also occurs sporadically in a variety of species (**Fig. 2**). Afflicted birds can be of any age, but most are 8 or more years old and many are more than 15 years old.[35,36] In one report, the incidence of atherosclerosis in the examined parrots was 91.9% in African grey parrots and 91.4% in Amazon parrots.[37] In birds older than 19 years, no unchanged vessels could be seen. The youngest bird with this alteration was 6 months

Table 1

Summary of disease conditions in older psittacines submitted to a private exotic species pathology service, ZEPS

Species	Total Number	Age Range	Average in the Range	Tumors	Chronic Liver Disease	Inflammatory Skin Lesions	Heart Lesions[a]	Gonadal Degeneration	Chronic Kidney Disease	Systemic Inflammation	Pneumoconiosis	Xanthoma
Budgerigar	229	6–15 y	7.8 y	153 (66.8%)	13 (5.7%)	8 (3.5%)	7 (3%)	10 (4.4%)	2 (0.9%)	18 (7.9%)	7 (3%)	5 (2.2%)
Lovebird	206	6–18 y	9.1 y	71 (34.4%)	21 (10%)	47 (22.8%)	23 (11.2%)	11 (5.3%)	0	18 (8.7%)	2 (1%)	5 (2.4%)
Amazon	168	30–86 y	38.2 y	59 (35%)	14 (8%)	10 (5.9%)	15 (8.9%)	5 (3%)	0	41 (24.4%)	15 (8.9%) (1 pulmonary fibrosis)	9 (5.3%)
Cockatiel	383	12–30 y	15.5 y	190 (49.6%)	40 (10%)	30 (7.8%)	33 (8.6%)	9 (2.3%)	22 (5.7%)	21 (5.5%)	9 (2.3%)	20 (5.2%)
Macaw	66	30–60 y	35 y	25 (37.8%)	5 (7.5%)	4 (6%)	10 (15%)	0	2 (3%)	14 (21.2%)	15 (22.7%)	2 (3%)
Cockatoo	27	30–45 y	34 y	8 (29.6%)	1 (3.7%)	3 (11%)	2 (7.4%)	0	1 (3.7%)	8 (29.6%)	0	1 (3.7%)
African grey	41	30–53 y	33 y	14 (34%)	3 (7.3%)	1 (2.4%)	8 (19.5%)	0	1 (2.4%)	8 (19.5%)	4 (9.7%)	0

[a] Heart lesions include artherosclerosis and/or lipofuscinosis.

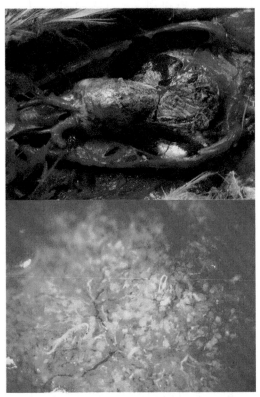

Fig. 1. (*Top*) Visceral gout associated with a chronic interstitial nephritis in a 31-year-old double yellow-headed Amazon (*Amazona oratrix magna*). (*Bottom*) In the close-up of the kidney, many uric acid tophi are visible.

old. The most affected groups with stage 2 to 4 lesions were the age groups with birds older than 26 years. One survey identified the average age as 12 years.[38]

The plaques can be found in the aorta, the brachiocephalic trunks, and the pectoral and carotid arteries. Coronary artery involvement is rare. Grossly, the arterial wall is

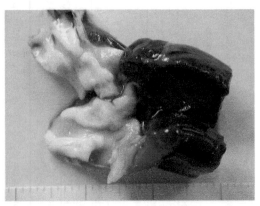

Fig. 2. Severe atherosclerosis of the larger arteries in a 25-year-old sulphur-crested cockatoo (*Cacatua galerita*).

variably thickened with roughened yellow intimal plaques. Histologically, atherosclerosis is characterized by vacuolated smooth muscle cells and macrophages (foam cells that contain cytoplasmic cholesterol and cholesterol esters) within the intimal layer of aorta and large arteries (**Fig. 3**). In addition, there can be microhemorrhage, chondroid metaplasia, fibrosis, and mineralization.[36,37] Commonly these lesions cause increased arterial resistance that affects the heart. Early changes in the heart include hypertrophy of the left ventricle followed by left ventricular dilation, dilation of the left atria, right heart dilation, and right heart failure. Right heart failure can lead to congestion, atrophy, and, subsequently, cirrhosis of the liver (**Fig. 4**). With these chronic changes, the birds may present with loss of body condition, although many die unexpectedly and are in excellent condition or even obese.

Many birds die because of a decreased blood supply to the brain as a result of severe narrowing of the carotid arteries. There may be a history of the bird going through periods of a loss of awareness of their surroundings in the days or weeks before their death.

Atherosclerosis can also lead to aneurysmal dilation of the arteries. It is rare to see ischemic disease of the heart.

Many risk factors have been postulated; increased age (adults) and a history of being fed a diet rich in fat are strongly associated with the condition.[36,38,39]

Lipofuscin

Another age-related lesion of the heart is the progressive accumulation of the cytoplasmic pigment lipofuscin. Lipofuscin is an intralysosomal pigment associated with excessive oxidation and polymerization of unsaturated fatty acids. It may accumulate in cells, including cardiac myocytes, secondary to a variety of disease processes, although it is usually associated with emaciation, chronic disease, or aging. It is usually considered an incidental necropsy finding. If severe, the myocardium may have a brown discoloration. Microscopically, fine yellow-brown pigment is seen, primarily near the cell nucleus, but more diffuse within the cytoplasm in severe cases.

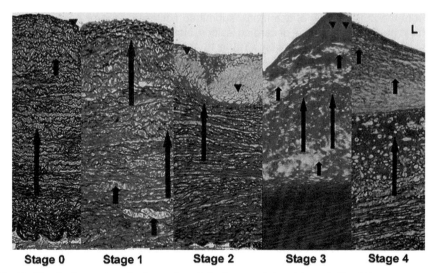

| Stage 0 | Stage 1 | Stage 2 | Stage 3 | Stage 4 |

Fig. 3. Histologic staging of atherosclerosis in the arteria brachiocephalica (elastica Weigert van Gieson staining). Arrowheads indicate intima. Large arrows indicate elastic fibers. Small arrows indicate interstitial matrix. L, lumen.

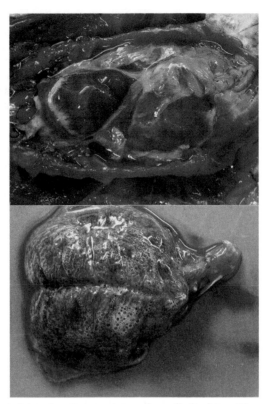

Fig. 4. Liver cirrhosis (*above*) and severe lung edema (*below*) in a 51-year-old African grey parrot (*P erithacus*).

From the ZEPS survey of commonly submitted psittacines examined, the species with the greatest percentage of cardiac lesions, including atherosclerosis or lipofuscinosis, were African grey parrots (see **Table 1**). Although only 41 birds were examined, 19.5%[8] of these birds had cardiac lesions. The next most common species with chronic heart lesions were macaws with 15% when examining 66 birds. Lovebirds surprisingly also had a significant amount of atherosclerosis and lipofuscinosis: Of 206 birds, 23 (11%) had cardiac lesions. Amazons, cockatiels, and cockatoos were identified with these lesions at 7% to 8.9% of the group. Only 3% of budgerigars, 7 out of 229, had heart lesions.

Integument

Aging changes in the skin of mammals (dogs and cats) are reported as a loss of elasticity, decreased pH, decreased hydration, decreased transepidermal water loss, and decreased skin-fold thickness.[40–42] Most studies in birds are of aging alterations of muscle and fat in the skin of commercially important food species (ie, geese, ducks, and poultry).[43–45]

One study in a group of aging macaws clinically noted degenerative changes of muscle wasting, weight loss, and decline in feather condition most prominent in birds over 40 years of age. The facial skin developed pigmented spots, polyps, and wartlike blemishes with cysts and wrinkling. Thinning of the skin was clinically evident on the face and feet of birds over 40 years of age.[46]

It could be postulated that increasing stiffness of joints and damage to the beak would affect feather grooming and subsequently the appearance of the feather coat (**Fig. 5**). However, no studies or reports are found that have identified such changes.

After cutaneous tumors, the most common primary skin lesion noted in the ZEPS survey of the lesions in aging psittacines was dermatitis. A number of the lesions seen were associated with a history of self-trauma, and an underlying cause was not always recognized (see **Table 1**). Lovebirds over the age of 6 had a significant percentage (22.8%) of inflammatory skin lesions. These primarily were the nonspecific syndrome of lovebird dermatitis, or chronic ulcerative dermatitis. The affected area was usually the patagium or neck and back, and apparent pruritis leads to self-mutilation. A viral cause has been suggested but has yet to be identified.[47] Only six of the inflammatory skin lesions were consistent with the syndrome polyfolliculitis. This is another skin lesion of which the cause is still unknown. Both of these syndromes are chronic and often recur.[47]

Liver

Chronic liver disease is the result of repeated injury to the liver over a lifetime. Unfortunately, by the time it has become an end-stage liver (cirrhosis/fibrosis), the identity of the injury can no longer be determined. The potential causes are numerous and can include toxicities (therapeutic agents or naturally occurring toxins); chronic cholangitis or obstructive biliary disease; chronic congestion from right-sided heart failure; disorders of metabolism, such as iron storage disease or hepatic lipidosis; and chronic hepatitis. These are the common insults for mammals and are also expected to be seen in birds.

The lesions of hepatic fibrosis, bile duct reduplication, and aggregates of granulocytic extramedullary hematopoiesis are the typical findings in chronic liver disease in birds.[48] Amazon parrots, cockatiels, macaws, and budgerigars seem to be more

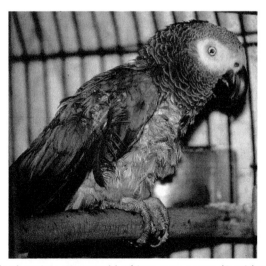

Fig. 5. Unkempt feathers in a 45-year-old African grey parrot (*P erithacus*). This bird had degenerative lesions of the joints in the wings and feet on physical examination and radiographically.

commonly recognized with chronic liver disease (**Fig. 6**).[49] Some cases also support inflammation of the liver and are described as chronic active hepatitis.

The cause of the changes is generally unknown. Cockatiels are reported to be sensitive to aflatoxins and it has been speculated that chronic active hepatitis in these birds may result from a previous exposure to aflatoxins.[49] Chlamydophila infections and exposure to bile-excreted toxins, such as Doxycycline, could also be potential causes.[49]

Grossly, the affected livers are variably shrunken, pale, and fibrotic. The capsule is often thickened and the edges of the liver are rounded (**Fig. 7**). In extreme cases, there may only be small firm nodules in place of the normal liver. Perihepatic effusion is common. The histologic appearance varies with the stage of the disease.[49]

A review of cases from the ZEPS survey found chronic liver disease in 7.5% to 10% of older lovebirds, Amazons, cockatiels, macaws, and African grey parrots. Budgerigars and cockatoos had the lowest percentage: 5.7% for budgerigars and 3.7% for cockatoos.

Musculoskeletal System

Degenerative lesions of the joints are not uncommon in older psittacine birds. Causes include previous trauma or infection, or metabolic conditions, such as gout. Grossly affected joints are enlarged, and there may be cartilagenous erosions. Cartilagenous flaps and free cartilage may be found in the joint cavity. Eventually, osteophytes and fibrosis form in the joint capsule and periarticular soft tissue.[50]

Degenerative changes of muscle wasting and joint stiffness were reported in a group of aging macaws and were most prominent birds over 40 years of age. Joint stiffness was characterized by a limitation in the range of motion of the joints, particularly the hock (intertarsal) joints. There were also twisting deformities that developed at the carpi, causing the primary flight feathers to twist laterally.[46]

Villonodular synovitis is a rarely described lesion of older cockatiels (Drury R. Reavill, DVM, PhD, personal observations). It appears as an inflammatory and proliferative process of the joint synovium. Until recently, these proliferative lesions were described as idiopathic and possibly immune mediated. They are now considered to be neoplastic.[51]

Reproductive System

Reproductive aging has been studied extensively in domestic species (poultry and quail). Generally, there is a decline in fertility and reproductive behavior. Gonadal function changes lead to the cessation of the ovulatory cycle and declining spermatogenesis. At the neuroendocrine level, age-related alterations affect the function of the gonadotropin-releasing hormone system.[52]

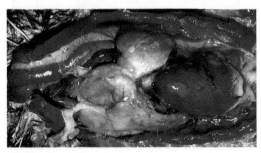

Fig. 6. Chronic liver disease in an Amazon parrot.

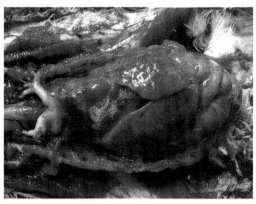

Fig. 7. Liver fibrosis in a 49-year-old Panama Amazon (*Amazona ochrocephala panamensis*).

There is one report on the reproductive life span of one group of free-flight breeding macaws (Parrot Jungle & Gardens, Homestead, FL, USA). The oldest birds to success-fully breed were 35 years old. It was noted that the average age for raising the first chicks was 13.5 years. The most productive years were from the late teens to the early twenties. In this group of birds, the reproductive activity declined in the twenties to thirties.[53]

Budgerigars and canaries (*Serinus canaria*) have reproductive life spans up to five times longer than comparatively sized mammals, such as rats and mice (4-5 years vs 1–2 years). In captivity under hospitable conditions, birds generally enjoy postre-productive life spans of one third or more of the total life span.[3]

Due to the seasonal variation in the size of the avian testis and presence or absence of spermatogenesis, changes in size of the testes or an absence of spermatogenesis must be carefully interpreted. Atrophy can be the end result of a degenerative process, and has been associated with generalized malnutrition, particularly vitamin E deficiency.[54]

Ovarian tumors are better reported in psittacines than are degenerative changes. In general, the ovary will support fewer primary ovarian follicles and these are usually small, degenerating structures (follicular atresia).

Examined cases from ZEPS identified gonadal degeneration evident in 4.4% of elderly budgerigars, 5.3% of lovebirds, 2.3% of cockatiels, and 3% of Amazon parrots (see **Table 1**).

Respiratory System

The effects of aging on the respiratory system in mammals are similar to those that occur in other organs: Maximum function gradually declines. Age-related changes in the lungs include decreases in the peak airflow, gas exchange, and vital capacity (the maximum amount of air that can be breathed out following a maximum inhalation); weakening of the respiratory muscles; and a decline in the effectiveness of lung defense mechanisms. In aging psittacines, problems found in the respiratory system are mostly related to repeated insults (and resulting inflammatory responses), such as inhalation of dusts, irritating gasses, and microorganisms, including viruses, bacteria, and fungal spores. These repeated "injuries" eventually lead to chronic scar tissue (fibrosis) and granulomatous changes. Also, circulatory and cardiac problems lead to (transient) interstitial edema that causes repeated minimal fibrotic reactions. The most commonly seen pathologic changes are chronic pulmonary interstitial fibrosis and focal granulomas with accumulation of dust-laden macrophages (pneumoconiosis or anthrasilicosis).

Chronic pulmonary interstitial fibrosis

Chronic pulmonary interstitial fibrosis has been more frequently described in the European population of older psittacines, although it is also been seen in the United States in a number of psittacines (Drury R. Reavill, DVM, PhD, personal observations). This syndrome was described in older Amazon parrots and is characterized as a chronic respiratory disease resulting in exercise intolerance. Pathologic examination revealed loss of functional lung tissue, pulmonary interstitial fibrosis, and right heart failure. Hematology revealed an elevated packed cell volume as a result of an increase in erythrocyte size and an increased hemoglobin mass per erythrocyte. In two patients, hypoxia and hypercapnia were demonstrated.[55] The cause of this syndrome was not identified but it was suggested that toxic substances, bacterial and chemical toxins, allergy, or viral infections could play a role in the pathogenesis of chronic pulmonary interstitial fibrosis in birds. In live birds, a computed tomography of the complete bird showed generalized lung alterations consistent with lung fibrosis. After taking lung biopsies, the tentative computed tomography diagnosis of pulmonary interstitial fibrosis was confirmed.[56]

Pneumoconiosis

Pneumoconiosis (anthrasilicosis) is the focal accumulation of dust-laden macrophages in the interatrial septa of the tertiary bronchi. These lesions generally suggest exposure to airborne pollutants and appear incidental in sedentary pet birds. The lungs may have macroscopic miliary black foci, although usually the accumulations are not observed grossly. The histiocytic aggregates are located subtending the mucosa of the epithelium of the air sacs, infundibula, and atria of tertiary bronchi, and around vessels. The histiocytes have intracytoplasmic granular black pigments and refractile pale yellow crystalline material, which is birefringent with polarized light. There may be infiltrates of lymphocytes and plasma cells associated with the nodules. When the crystalline material has been examined by transmission electron microscopy and x-ray spectra, most of the crystals are silicates. The silicates do not appear to elicit fibrosis in birds.[57]

SPECIAL SENSES

Cataracts are common lesions described in older animals. Acquired cataracts have been associated with nutritional deficiencies, trauma, toxins, infection and inflammation of the eye, and aging. Many older psittacine birds have cataracts and falcons appear to have a higher incidence than many other birds. Cataracts are opacities of the lens secondary to altered lens metabolism, usually following some injury to lens epithelium or capsule (epithelial basement membrane). Cataracts can be classified according to age of onset or location within the lens. Morphologically the usual structure of the capsule and lens fibers is altered.

Grossly, cataracts present as lens opacities. Histologic early changes may be limited to swelling of lens fibers with bladder cell formation. There may be epithelial hyperplasia as well as foci of capsular thinning. With progression, cystoid spaces can develop and lens protein will coagulate and fibers fragment. Mature cataracts involve the entire lens. Hypermature cataracts develop when necrotic cortical material is lost, leading to a small lens with a wrinkled capsule.[58,59]

In a group of aging macaws with ophthalmic disorders, cataracts were the most common problem. These would initially present as an opaque striation in the lens cortex. Birds with rapidly developing cataracts often progressed to phacolytic uveitis and, if left untreated, became blind.[46]

Nervous System

Degenerative aging changes of the central nervous system are best characterized in humans. Few articles cover degenerative lesions in the avian brain. These include studies about song-learning of various species, amyloid plaques in a woodpecker, and atherosclerosis in quail.[60–62] Specifically in psittacines, lipofuscin, atherosclerosis, and Lafora bodies have been described.[63–65]

Lipofuscin is a common finding in the neural cell bodies of older parrots. Generally, the lesion is mild, but in some birds the accumulation can be prominent. It is suspected that in most cases this pigment accumulation does not have a functional significance.[66]

Atherosclerosis of the carotid arteries and even involvement of the cerebral arteries may result in cerebral ischemia and hypertension.[64]

Lafora bodies may not necessarily be lesions of aging. One investigator (Drury R. Reavill, DVM, PhD, personal observations) has identified it only rarely (blue-headed pionus [*Pionus menstruus*], blue-fronted Amazon, cockatiel) and all have been adult birds. Clinically, it is characterized by tremors, ataxia, or seizures. Lafora disease is characterized by periodic acid-Schiff–positive polyglycosan inclusions (Lafora bodies) found in neurons and muscle. Polyglycosan differs from normal glycogen in being short-chained, densely packed, insoluble, and heavily phosphorylated.[65]

Oncology

Age has an important influence on the likelihood of tumor development. This is due to an increase in genetic damage from the action of environmental agents and errors in repair. Few studies have reviewed numerous tumors and their biologic features, including the age of the birds at diagnosis (**Fig. 8**).

Air sac carcinomas

Air sac carcinomas are rare tumors and it is often difficult to definitively identify the air sac as the tissue of origin. The few cases described have been in mature, large psittacines (cockatoo, African grey parrot, macaw, Amazon parrot).[63,67,68] Cases were initially presented with cystic masses or bony lesions primarily involving the humerus.

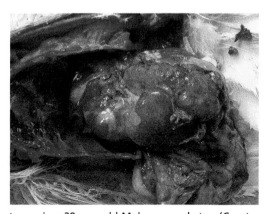

Fig. 8. Cystic ovary tumor in a 28-year-old Moluccan cockatoo (*Cacatua moluccensis*).

Hemangiomas and hemangiosarcomas

Hemangiomas are benign tumors of vascular endothelium. They are reported more commonly in budgerigars than in other birds and usually occur in the skin (feet, inguinal region, cloaca, side of neck, wing) and spleen. The average age of occurrence is 10.8 years (range 3–20 years).[69]

Hemangiosarcoma is the malignant form of hemangioma, also known as malignant hemangioendothelioma or angiosarcoma. The beak, wings, feet, legs, and cloaca are the most common sites for cutaneous hemangiosarcomas. Cockatiels lead the list of affected species, which also include chickens (*Gallus gallus domesticus*), swans (*Cygnus* sp), Amazon parrots, lovebirds, African grey parrots, pionus parrots, budgerigars, parakeets, canaries, and finches. Hemangiosarcomas are locally invasive and multicentric. Skin tumors tend to appear inflamed and necrotic. The affected age range is similar to that of hemangiomas and the sexes are evenly represented.[70]

Hemangiolipomas, benign tumors of adipose tissue and blood vessels, are uncommon tumors that originate in the subcutaneous tissue on the body or limbs. Affected species include a budgerigar, a yellow-collared macaw (*Primolius auricollis*), a cockatiel, a lovebird, a blue-fronted Amazon, and a canary. All affected birds were more than 9 years of age.[70]

Myelolipomas, uncommon tumors, are well-delineated, expansile, benign extramarrow neoplasms composed of varying proportions of fat and hematopoietic cells. They are considered choristomatous (histologically normal tissue in an abnormal location) hematopoietic stem cell elements. According to the literature, the majority occur on the wings (some bilaterally) of adult (7–20 years old) female cockatiels. In lovebirds, myelolipomas occur as multiple masses in the subcutaneous tissues of the body and wing.[70–72]

Reproductive tumors

Seminomas, tumors of immature germ cells, grossly appear yellow-red and cause enlargement of the testis. Anorexia, lethargy, and dyspnea were the most common clinical signs reported. The average age at diagnosis was 9.2 years from one study.[73]

Sertoli cell tumors are primary testicular tumors of gonadal-stroma that arise from the Sertoli (sustentacular) cells. Sertoli cell tumors are generally firm, gray-white neoplasms that appear nodular on section. The common clinical signs reported included anorexia, dyspnea, cardiac changes (bradycardia, murmur) and, in budgerigars, a color change of the cere from blue to brown. The average age at diagnosis was 10.2 years in one study.[73]

Xanthomas

Xanthomas are not true neoplasms, but they are locally invasive and are usually identified in older psittacines. The average age of affected birds is 10 years (range 3–30 years). These are masses of foamy macrophages, multinucleated giant cells, and cholesterol clefts that produce thickened, dimpled skin with yellow to orange coloration and occur infrequently in internal organs.[69]

A review of case submissions of older psittacines to ZEPS identified older budgerigars as having an increased number of tumors (66.7%). Tumors on cockatiels were identified in about half of the cases. Tumors in the other species—lovebirds, Amazons, macaws, cockatoos, and African greys—comprised about one third of the case submissions.

SUMMARY

Aging processes leading to specific organ problems are not obvious in aging psittacines. In general, birds live long and age slowly, despite their high metabolic rates and very high total lifetime energy expenditures. Most pathologic processes seen in older parrots are generally not specific for aging because they are seen in young birds as well. Pathologic processes that have a tendency to occur more in older psittacines are atherosclerosis and repeated injury processes, such as chronic pulmonary interstitial fibrosis, pneumoconiosis, liver fibrosis, and lens cataracts. Also some neoplasms are more often seen at an older age.

REFERENCES

1. Holmes DJ. Naturally long-lived animal models for the study of slow aging and longevity. Ann N Y Acad Sci 2004;1019:483–5.
2. Holmes DJ, Kristan DM. Comparative and alternative approaches and novel animal models for aging research: introduction to special issue. Age (Dordr) 2008;30:63–73.
3. Holmes DJ, Ottinger MA. Birds as long-lived animal models for the study of aging. Exp Gerontol 2003;38:1365–75.
4. Holmes DJ, Ottinger MA. Domestic and wild birds models for studying aging. Chapter 30. In: Conn PM, editor. Handbook of models for human aging. Amsterdam, Boston: Elsevier Academic Press; 2006. p. 350–63.
5. Møller AP. Relative longevity and field metabolic rate in birds. J Evol Biol 2008;21: 1379–86.
6. Holmes DJ, Austad SN. Birds as animal models for the comparative biology of aging: a prospectus. J Gerontol A Biol Sci Med Sci 1995;50:B59–66.
7. Holmes DJ, Flückiger R, Austad SN. Comparative biology of aging in birds: an update. Exp Gerontol 2001;36:869–83.
8. Ogburn CE, Carlberg K, Ottinger MA, et al. Exceptional cellular resistance to oxidative damage in long-lived birds requires active gene expression. J Gerontol A Biol Sci Med Sci 2001;56:B468–74.
9. Harman D. Prolongation of life: role of free radical reactions in aging. J Am Geriatr Soc 1969;17:721–35.
10. Cerami A. Accumulation of advanced glycosylation endproducts on proteins and nucleic acids: role in ageing. Prog Clin Biol Res 1985;195:79–90.
11. Kristal BS, Yu BP. An emerging hypothesis: synergistic induction of aging by free radicals and Maillard reactions. J Gerontol 1992;47:B107–14.
12. Barja G. Mitochondrial free radical production and aging in mammals and birds. Ann N Y Acad Sci 1998;854:224–38.
13. Barja G. Mitochondrial oxygen consumption and reactive oxygen species production are independently modulated: implications for aging studies. Rejuvenation Res 2007;10:215–24.
14. Del Maestro RF. An approach to free radicals in medicine and biology. Acta Physiol Scandia 1980;492:153–68.
15. Monnier VM, Sell DR, Ramanakoppa HN, et al. Mechanisms of protection against damage mediated by the Maillard reaction in aging. Gerontology 1991;37: 152–65.
16. Monnier VM, Fogarty JF, Monnier C, et al. Glycation, glycoxidation, and other Maillard reaction products. In: Yu BP, editor. Methods in aging research. Boca Raton (FL): CRC; 1999. p. 657–81.

17. Kirkwood TB, Holliday R. The evolution of ageing and longevity. Proc R Soc Lond B Biol Sci 1979;205:531–46.
18. Sozou PD, Kirkwood TB. A stochastic model of cell replicative senescence based on telomere shortening, oxidative stress, and somatic mutations in nuclear and mitochondrial DNA. J Theor Biol 2001;213:573–86.
19. Proctor CJ, Kirkwood TB. Modelling telomere shortening and the role of oxidative stress. Mech Ageing Dev 2002;123:351–63.
20. Kirkwood TB. Understanding the odd science of aging. Cell 2005;120:437–47.
21. Cotran RS, Kumar V, Collins. Cellular pathology II: adaptations, intracellular accumulations, and cell aging. In: Cotran RS, Kumar V, Collins T, editors. Robbins pathologic basis of disease. Philadelphia: WB Saunders Co; 1999. p. 31–49.
22. Finkel T, Holbrook NJ. Oxidants, oxidative stress and the biology of ageing. Nature 2000;408:239–47.
23. Melov S, Ravenscroft J, Malik S, et al. Extension of life-span with superoxide dismutase/catalase mimetics. Science 2000;289:1567–9.
24. Harley CB, Villeponteau B. Telomeres and telomerase in aging and cancer. Curr Opin Genet Dev 1995;249–55.
25. Harley CB. Telomerase therapeutics for degenerative diseases. Curr Mol Med 2005;5:205–11.
26. Swanberg SE, Delaney ME. Telomeres and aging: birds. Chapter 29. In: Conn PM, editor. Handbook of models for human aging. Amsterdam, Boston: Elsevier Academic Press; 2006. p. 339–49.
27. Delany ME, Krupkin AB, Miller MM. Organization of telomere sequences in birds: evidence for arrays of extreme length and for in vivo shortening. Cytogenet Cell Genet 2000;90:139–45.
28. Delany ME, Daniels LM, Swanberg SE, et al. Telomeres in the chicken: genome stability and chromosome ends. Poult Sci 2003;82:917–26.
29. Hausmann MF, Winkler DW, O'Reilly KM, et al. Telomeres shorten more slowly in long-lived birds and mammals than in short-lived ones. Proc R Soc Lond B Biol Sci 2003;270:1387–92.
30. Haussmann MF, Winkler DW, Huntington CE, et al. Telomerase activity is maintained throughout the lifespan of long-lived birds. Exp Gerontol 2007;42:610–8.
31. Salomons HM, Mulder GA, van de Zande L, et al. Telomere shortening and survival in free-living corvids. Proc Biol Sci 2009;276:3157–65.
32. Perry RA. The avian patient. In: Ritchie BW, Harrison GJ, Harrison LR, editors. Avian medicine: principles and application. Lake Worth (FL): Wingers Publishing, Inc; 1994. p. 30.
33. Spadafori G, Speer BL. Birds for dummies. Foster City (CA): IDG Books Worldwide, Inc; 1999. p. 275–82.
34. Pees M, Krautwald-Junghanns ME. Cardiovascular physiology and diseases of pet birds. Vet Clin North Am Exot Anim Pract 2009;12:81–97.
35. Phalen DN, Hays HB, Filippich LJ, et al. Heart failure in a macaw with atherosclerosis of the aorta and brachiocephalic arteries. J Am Vet Med Assoc 1996;209:1435–40.
36. Schmidt RE, Reavill DR, Phalen DN. 1. Cardiovascular system. In: Schmidt R, Reavill D, Phalen D, editors. Pathology of pet and aviary birds. Ames (IA): Iowa State Press; 2003. p. 3–16.
37. Fricke C, Schmidt V, Cramer K, et al. Characterization of atherosclerosis by histochemical and immunohistochemical methods in African grey parrots (*Psittacus erithacus*) and Amazon parrots (*Amazona* spp. Avian Dis 2009;53:466–72.

38. Garner MM, Raymond JT. A retrospective study of atherosclerosis in birds. In: Association of Avian Veterinarians Annual Conference Proceedings; Pittsburgh (PA); 2003. p. 59–66.
39. Bavelaar FJ, Beynen AC. Atherosclerosis in parrots. A review. Vet Q 2004;26: 50–60.
40. Young LA, Dodge JC, Guest KJ, et al. Age, breed, sex and period effects on skin biophysical parameters for dogs fed canned dog food. J Nutr 2002;132:1695S–7S.
41. Cline J, Young L, Kerr W, et al. Effect of age and sex on feline skin. Nestle purina nutrition forum 2003, Poster presentation.
42. Pageon H, Asselineau D. An in vitro approach to the chronological aging of skin by glycation of the collagen: the biological effect of glycation on the reconstructed skin model. Ann N Y Acad Sci 2005;1043:529–32.
43. Bochno R, Brzozowski W, Murawska D. Age-related changes in the distribution of lean, fat with skin and bones in duck carcasses. Br Poult Sci 2005;46:199–203.
44. Bochno R, Murawska D, Brzostowska U. Age-related changes in the distribution of lean fat with skin and bones in goose carcasses. Poult Sci 2006;85:1987–91.
45. Christensen KD, Zimmermann NG, Wyatt CL, et al. Dietary and environmental factors affecting skin strength in broiler chickens. Poult Sci 1994;73:224–35.
46. Clubb SL, Karpinski L. Aging in macaws. J Assoc Avian Vet 1993;7:31–3.
47. Schmidt RE, Lightfoot TL. Integument. Chapter 13. In: Harrison GJ, Lightfoot TL, editors. Clinical avian medicine—volume I. Palm Beach (FL): Spix Publishing, Inc; 2006. p. 395–409.
48. Clyde VL, Orosz SE, Munson L. Severe hepatic fibrosis and bile duct hyperplasia in four Amazon parrots. J Av Med Surg 1996;10:252–7.
49. Schmidt RE, Reavill DR, Phalen D. Liver. Chapter 4. In: Schmidt R, Reavill D, Phalen D, editors. Pathology of pet and aviary birds. Ames (IA): Iowa State Press; 2003b. p. 67–95.
50. Schmidt RE, Reavill DR, Phalen D. Musculoskeltal system. Chapter 9. In: Schmidt R, Reavill D, Phalen D, editors. Pathology of pet and aviary birds. Ames (IA): Iowa State Press; 2003c. p. 149–64.
51. Perka C, Labs K, Zippel H, et al. Localized pigmented villonodular synovitis of the knee joint: neoplasm or reactive granuloma? A review of 18 cases. Rheumatology (Oxford) 2000;39(2):172–8.
52. Ottinger MA, Wu J, Pelican K. Neuroendocrine regulation of reproduction in birds and clinical applications of GnRH analogues in birds and mammals. Seminars in Avian and Exotic Pet Medicine 2006;11:71–9.
53. Schubot RM, Clubb KJ, Clubb SL. Psittacine aviculture. Prospectives, techniques, and research. Loxahatchee (FL): Avicuitural Breeding and Research Center; 1992.
54. Schmidt RE, Reavill DR, Phalen D. Reproductive system. In: Schmidt R, Reavill D, Phalen D, editors. Pathology of pet and aviary birds. Ames (IA): Iowa State Press; 2003d. Chapter 6, p. 109–20.
55. Zandvliet MMJM, Dorrestein GM, van der Hage M. Chronic pulmonary interstitial fibrosis in Amazon parrots. Avian Pathol 2001;30:517–24.
56. Amann O, Kik MJL, Passon-Vastenburg MHAC, et al. Chronic pulmonary interstitial fibrosis in a blue-fronted Amazon parrot (*Amazona aestiva aestiva*). Avian Dis 2007;51:150–3.
57. Schmidt RE, Reavill DR, Phalen D. Respiratory system. In: Schmidt R, Reavill D, Phalen D, editors. Pathology of pet and aviary birds. Ames (IA): Iowa State Press; 2003e. Chapter 2, p. 17–40.

58. Tsai SS, Park JH, Hirai K, et al. Eye lesions in pet birds. Avian Pathol 1993;22: 95–112.
59. Brooks DE. Avian cataracts. Seminars in Avian and Exotic Pet Medicine 1997;6: 131–7.
60. Nakayama H, Katayama K, Ikawa A, et al. Cerebral amyloid angiopathy in an aged great spotted woodpecker (*Picoides major*). Neurobiol Aging 1999;20: 53–6.
61. Brainard MS, Doupe AJ. Postlearning consolidation of birdsong: stabilizing effects of age and anterior forebrain lesions. J Neurosci 2001;21:2501–17.
62. Hoekstra KA, Velleman SG. Brain microvascular and intracranial artery resistance to atherosclerosis is associated with heme oxygenase and ferritin in Japanese quail. Mol Cell Biochem 2008;307:1–12.
63. Schmidt RE, Reavill DR, Phalen D. Nervous System. Chapter 10. In: Schmidt R, Reavill D, Phalen D, editors. Pathology of pet and aviary birds. Ames (IA): Iowa State Press; 2003f. p. 165–76.
64. Jones MP, Orosz SE. Overview of avian neurology and neurological diseases. Seminars in Avian and Exotic Pet Medicine 1996;5(3):150–64.
65. Britt JO Jr, Paster MB, Gonzales C, et al. Lafora body neuropathy in a cockatiel. Companion Anim Pract 1989;19:31–3.
66. Reece RL, Macwhirter P. Neuronal ceroid lipofuscinosis in a lovebird. Vet Rec 1988;122:187.
67. Powers LV, Merrill CL, Degernes LA, et al. Axillary cystadenocarcinoma in a Moluccan cockatoo (Cacatua moluccensis). Avian Dis 1998;42:408–12.
68. Radial SR, Shearer PL, Butler R, et al. Airsac cystadenocarcinomas in cockatoos. Aust Vet J 2007;84:213–6.
69. Reavill DR. Tumors of pet birds. Vet Clin Exot Anim 2004;7:537–60.
70. Reavill DR. Pet bird oncology. Proceedings of the Association of Avian Veterinarians conference, Avian Specialty Advanced Program, Orlando (FL); 2001. p. 29–43.
71. Andreasen JR, Andreasen CB, Latimer KL, et al. Thoracoabdominal myelolipomas and carcinoma in a lovebird (*Agapornis*) sp. J Vet Diagn Invest 1995;7: 271–2.
72. Latimer KS, Rakich PM. Subcutaneous and hepatic myelolipomas in four exotic birds. Vet Pathol 1995;32:84–7.
73. Reavill D, Echols MS, Schmidt R. Testicular tumors of 54 birds and therapy in 6 cases. In: Proceedings of the Association of Avian Veterinarians; 2004. p. 335–7.

Index

Note: Page numbers of article titles are in **boldface** type.

A

Vet Clin Exot Anim 13 (2010) 151–169
doi:10.1016/S1094-9194(10)00009-5
1094-9194/10/$ – see front matter © 2010 Elsevier Inc. All rights reserved.

Moving?

Make sure your subscription moves with you!

To notify us of your new address, find your **Clinics Account Number** (located on your mailing label above your name), and contact customer service at:

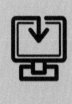

Email: journalscustomerservice-usa@elsevier.com

800-654-2452 (subscribers in the U.S. & Canada)
314-447-8871 (subscribers outside of the U.S. & Canada)

Fax number: 314-447-8029

Elsevier Health Sciences Division
Subscription Customer Service
3251 Riverport Lane
Maryland Heights, MO 63043

*To ensure uninterrupted delivery of your subscription, please notify us at least 4 weeks in advance of move.

Printed and bound by CPI Group (UK) Ltd, Croydon, CR0 4YY

18/10/2024

01775924-0001